Green Smoothies for Life

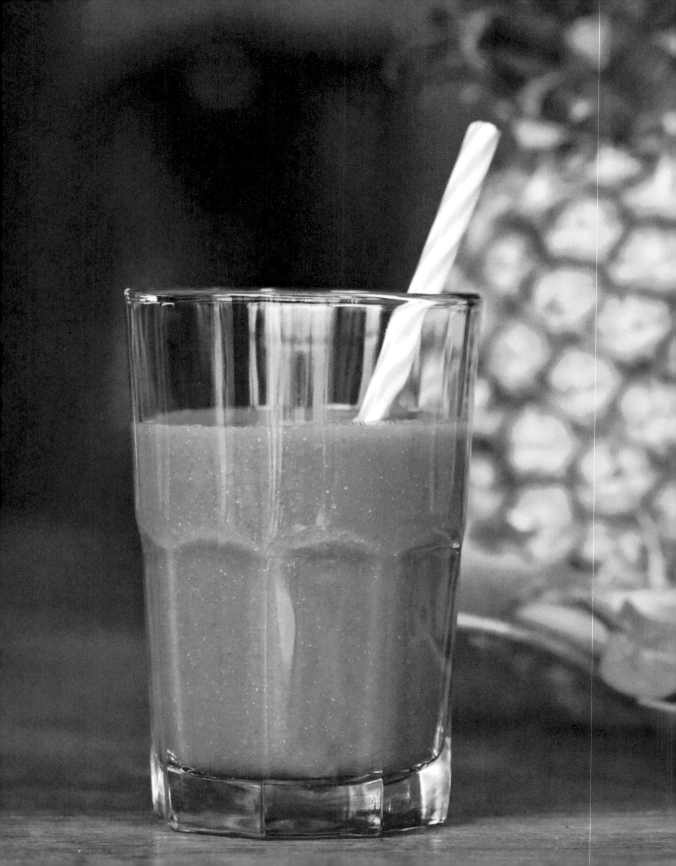

Green Smoothies For Life

JJ SMITH

ATRIA PAPERBACK

NEW YORK   LONDON   TORONTO   SYDNEY   NEW DELHI

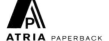

ATRIA PAPERBACK

Atria Books
An Imprint of Simon & Schuster, Inc.
1230 Avenue of the Americas
New York, NY 10020

First Atria Paperback edition December 2016

ATRIA PAPERBACK and colophon are trademarks of Simon & Schuster, Inc.

For information about special discounts for bulk purchases, please contact Simon & Schuster Special Sales at 1-866-506-1949 or business@simonandschuster.com.

The Simon & Schuster Speakers Bureau can bring authors to your live event. For more information or to book an event, contact the Simon & Schuster Speakers Bureau at 1-866-248-3049 or visit our website at www.simonspeakers.com.

Manufactured in the United States of America

10 9 8

Library of Congress Cataloging-in-Publication Data is available.

ISBN 978-1-5011-0065-9
ISBN 978-1-5011-0066-6 (ebook)

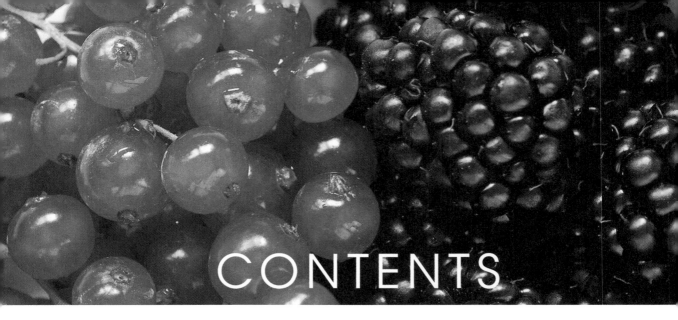

CONTENTS

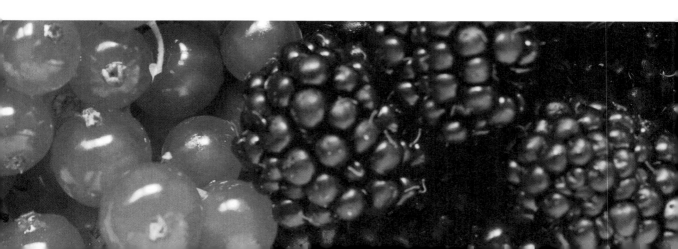

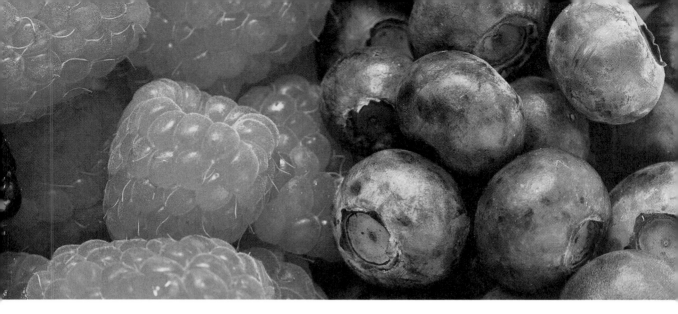

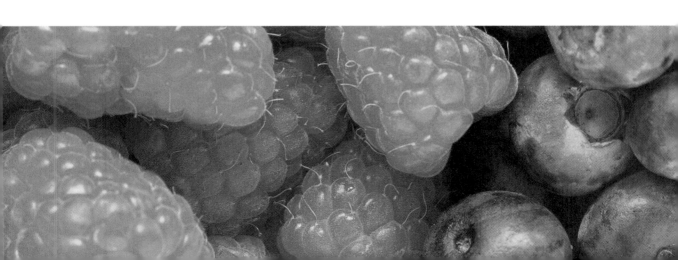

IMPORTANT NOTE TO READERS

The information contained in this book is for your education. It is not intended to diagnose, treat, or cure any medical condition or dispense medical advice. If you decide to follow my plan, you should seek the advice and counsel of your licensed health professional and then use your own judgment.

It is important to obtain proper medical advice before you make any decisions about nutrition, diet, supplements, or other health-related issues that are discussed in this book. Neither the author nor the publisher is qualified to provide medical, financial, or psychological advice or services. The reader should consult an appropriate health-care professional before heeding any of the advice given in this book.

INTRODUCTION

What an amazing journey this has been. Green smoothies have taken the world by storm over the last few years, and I am honored to be a part of such a great movement. A few years ago, I introduced the 10-Day Green Smoothie Cleanse to the world, and as a result, millions of people have been using green smoothies to not only detoxify and lose weight but also to improve their health and get their sexy back, some say for the first time in years. The 10-Day Green Smoothie Cleanse changes your eating habits, helps you get rid of cravings for sweets, and reprograms your cravings toward healthier foods instead. But you can't keep repeating the cleanse over and over. Ideally, there would be a way to incorporate the green smoothie philosophy into a more permanent meal plan. The goal of *Green Smoothies for Life* is to do just that.

In the pages that follow, I show you how to detox your body, lose weight permanently, and achieve great health. On this 30-Day Program, you will enjoy delicious green smoothies, hot meals, snacks, and desserts that will nourish every cell in your body so that you not only get slim but healthy and vibrant as well. You will give your body the quality nutrition it needs while cleansing your cells and internal organs. Your skin will become brighter, your eyes will become whiter, your hair will get shinier, and your overall look will be more youthful and radiant!

After the thirty days, you will never have to go on a diet again. A typical diet is something you do for a specified period of time. What usually happens when you "go off" the diet? You gain all the weight back. With this 30-Day Program, we are going to retrain your taste buds to desire and crave healthier foods so you never have to think about dieting again. You can achieve this without counting calories or points, or measuring portion sizes, or eating bland, packaged foods. Your body will begin to naturally crave and desire healthy, natural foods.

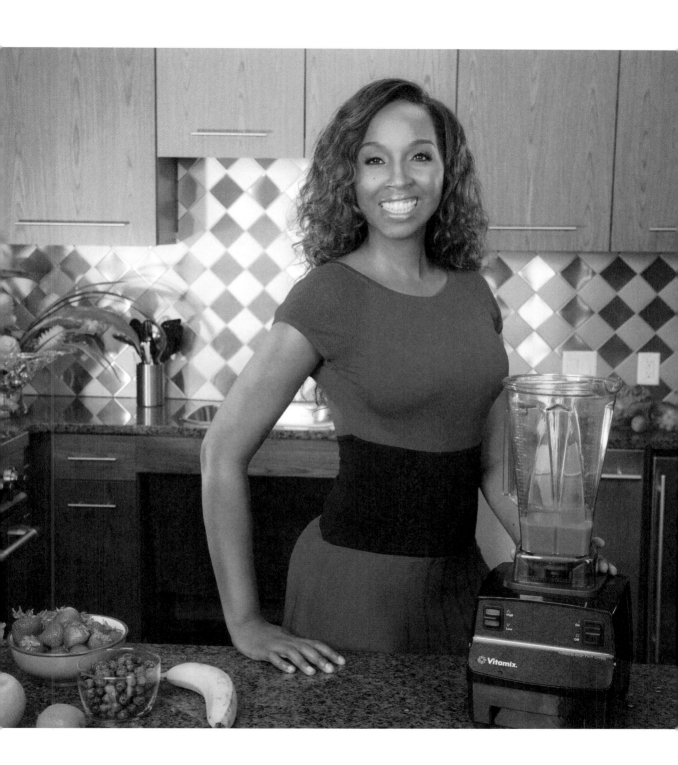

WHAT YOU CAN EXPECT:

- Lose up to 20 pounds in 30 days
- Detox while eating hot, healthy meals every day
- Increase energy and regain a second youth
- Reduce cravings for sugar, pastas, and bread
- Sleep more restfully
- Experience better digestion and less bloating, leading to a slimmer waistline.

This plan offers you a permanent solution that can help you create and live your best life. Maybe you have had some success in the past, but you still haven't reached your goal weight. It's time to commit to this program that has given others the results they desired.

You have a desire to upgrade your life, improve your heath, and live better. You may have made excuses in the past, but now something deep inside you is whispering, or maybe even shouting, that the time to make a change is NOW. Know that anything you desire, you can create in your life, including the body of your dreams. You just have to commit and decide that the time is NOW. Deep down, you know it's time to upgrade your life.

You've decided to embark on this 30-day journey because you want more out of your life, and you deserve it. Don't be afraid, as I will be here to support and cheer you on through our Green Smoothie Facebook group.

Millions Have Joined the Green Smoothie Movement

A few years ago, after years of clean, healthy eating and detoxing, I was bedridden with mercury poisoning from my silver dental fillings! I had high levels of mercury in my brain, gut, liver, and kidneys. I couldn't get out of bed for two months. And when I did, just making the bed required that I lie back down to rest! My health, energy, and motivation were at an all-time low.

After a long and slow recovery, I decided I needed to do something to get my health and energy back, as well as lose the 20 pounds I had gained while bedridden. After learning how raw greens can heal the body, I created the 10-Day Green Smoothie Cleanse.

Already an advocate of detoxing, I also knew I needed to rid my body of excess waste and toxins that had accumulated as a result of the mercury poisoning.

Once I created the 10-Day Green Smoothie Cleanse, I asked my community of friends and family if they would join and support me. My goal was to get 10 people to say yes. I was pleasantly surprised to find that about 100 of them wanted to do it! We created a Facebook group to keep one another motivated. Because the results, which we shared with pictures and testimonials, were so phenomenal, in less than two months about 10,000 people joined the Facebook group and committed to doing the cleanse with us. In just 10 days, folks were losing 10 to 15 pounds, getting energized, reversing health conditions, and feeling better than they had in years.

When I completed my first cleanse, I lost 11 pounds. My energy was high, my skin was radiant, and my digestion had improved and the bloating had dissipated. I felt renewed and motivated again! Before I began the cleanse, I had been taking twenty-four supplements a day to help my body recover from mercury poisoning. Since completing the cleanse, I have been taking only four supplements per day and have such a positive outlook on my health that I now have the energy to focus on my life dreams and goals. I learned that green smoothies are a great way to give the body the proper nutrition not only to keep it healthy and vibrant but also to nourish the spark of life within it.

Fast-forward to today, 2 million pounds have been lost on the green smoothie cleanse, which I codified into a book, the #1 *New York Times* bestseller *The 10-Day Green Smoothie Cleanse*. The book's techniques are so successful and the word of mouth about the diet so organic, the book has stayed on the *New York Times* bestseller list for more than fifty-two consecutive weeks, and we now have over 1 million followers/fans. Now, the number one question we get is: *What do I do after the 10-day cleanse?* The 30-Day Program is the answer to that.

The 10-Day Green Smoothie Cleanse is a great way to detox and jump-start weight loss; the 30-Day Program allows you to continue and maintain your weight loss. After the 10-day cleanse, you can use this book to continue the success that you have achieved. This book provides a 30-day meal plan and new recipes. It is a long-term eating plan that you can maintain for life. The 30-Day Program will go much further to help you establish new habits to ensure you achieve your long-term weight-loss goals.

The 30-Day Program teaches you how to use green smoothies and clean eating to lose weight permanently. In addition to providing new green smoothie recipes, it teaches you how to incorporate healthy, clean meals into your diet, how to snack, and even incorporate desserts into your regimen. This is truly a plan you can maintain for life.

What's in This Book?

PART 1 provides a sample meal plan, with 30 days of green smoothie recipes, hot meal recipes, snacks, and desserts. It includes a step-by-step prescriptive regimen for you to follow each day, along with the shopping lists, recipes, guidelines, FAQs, and more. You'll be surprised to find that your body will begin to crave healthy foods, allowing you to easily follow this program. All you'll need to do is follow the guidelines for each day, and listen to your body, which will reward you for your efforts.

PART 2 provides information about twenty-one detox methods (several of which have not been previously discussed in my other books), along with their benefits, cost, expected results, and completion time. The costs range from just a few dollars and include ingredients you can get at your local grocer to several hundreds of dollars for machines and treatments that assist in detoxifying the body. These twenty-one methods are used by my VIP members (see Appendix B) and are tried-and-true methods that folks enjoy incorporating into their regimen.

PART 3 offers a little extra motivation with several success stories of individuals who have used green smoothies and clean eating to achieve weight-loss success. These stories will help you see that you can have success too. People just like you have had extraordinary success. These individuals have all lost 40 or more pounds and have kept the weight off by incorporating green smoothies and healthy, clean meals into their regimen. You can read their stories, told in their own words, along with their before and after pictures.

PART 4 will provide a primer on the DHEMM (Detox/Hormonal Balance/Eat Clean/ Mental Mastery/Move) System and share details on where to get more information on it. Years ago, I revolutionized the weight-loss industry with the DHEMM System, an approach to long-term weight loss, including advanced topics like balancing hormones for weight loss. This section introduces you to my DHEMM philosophy.

● ● ●

The 30-Day Program is a blueprint that will allow you to discover a path to losing weight once and for all. It's a whole new way of living and enjoying foods. Over the past few years, I've found that the secret to losing weight is not about avoiding foods, but enjoying foods. The next 30 days will challenge you, but you will find it to be an incredibly rewarding experience. You will begin to feel good in your own skin and feel better than ever about yourself and your body.

To summarize, throughout this book, you will read about the following programs by JJ:

- *10-Day Green Smoothie Cleanse (10-Day GSC):* Most people jump-start their weight loss with the 10-Day Green Smoothie Cleanse. There is a full and modified version of this cleanse to provide you with two options that best fit your goals and lifestyle. The full cleanse consists of three green smoothies and snacks for 10 days, while the modified cleanse consists of two green smoothies, a healthy dinner and snacks for 10 days.

- *Green Smoothies for Life (30-Day Program):* After you complete the 10 days, folks transition to Green Smoothies for Life. They use the 30-Day Program to learn to incorporate green smoothies into their daily regimen for continued weight loss and maintenance and improved overall health. But the smoothies are only part of the mosaic. Hot meats, snacks, and even desserts are also part of the program. This book will focus on the details of how to use the 30-Day Program to meet your long-term weight-loss goals.

- **DHEMM System:** The DHEMM System is the most comprehensive approach to weight loss that will not only ensure that you lose the weight, but that you keep it off as well. As you look to maintain your weight loss, the DHEMM System provides all the advanced approaches to weight loss that are commonly overlooked by traditional dieting, including detoxing and balancing your hormones for weight loss. In the DHEMM Primer in this book, you'll receive an overview of the DHEMM System.

● ● ●

Congratulations on taking control of your health by caring for your body and feeding it what it needs to be slim, healthy, and vibrant!

Know that you are a person who can change. You can have a much better life than you have right now. Imagine going shopping and enjoying the way clothes look on your new body. Imagine having so much energy that you look forward to working out. Imagine feeling in total control of your life and your eating decisions. Imagine having the energy to rekindle your love life. Imagine finally having the confidence to achieve dreams you once thought were impossible; to go after that promotion you deserve or start your very own business. All of these things and so much more are waiting for you. We are surrounded by so many unhealthy food choices that are enticing and addictive. But with this 30-Day Program, you can leave old eating habits behind and establish new, healthier eating habits. I know how much courage it takes to begin a new life and a new relationship with food. I support you and encourage you in your efforts. And if you need support, join our Facebook Group at https://www.facebook.com/groups/Green.Smoothie.Cleanse.

Tips for Success with Green Smoothies

Green smoothies are loaded with beneficial vitamins, minerals, antioxidants, anti-inflammatory substances, phytonutrients, fiber, water, and more! They are also stuffed with chlorophyll, which is similar in structure to the hemoglobin in human blood. So drinking green smoothies is much like receiving a cleansing blood transfusion. Despite their simplicity, green smoothies provide a ton of nutritional benefits that lead to a healthier lifestyle. These benefits include weight loss, increased energy, reduction in food cravings, clearer skin, and much more.

THREE HEALTH-TRANSFORMING BENEFITS OF GREEN SMOOTHIES

1. *Eliminate Cravings for Unhealthy Foods.* Green smoothies help reduce and, over time, eliminate your cravings for unhealthy foods. Green smoothies contain fiber, healthy fats, and protein, all of which help to slow down the digestion and absorption of sugar. This will keep your blood sugar steady so you don't have blood sugar highs and lows that result in cravings for sweet, sugary foods. Green smoothies help return the body to a more natural state of health, feeling energized, satisfied, and cravings-free.

2. *Vibrant, Radiant Health.* I believe that natural, healthy eating is the secret to inner and outer beauty. When you eat natural, whole foods, you simply look and feel better and younger. Once you eat in a manner that keeps your cells clean and healthy, you will begin to look radiant, despite your age. When you start drinking green smoothies, one of the first places where you'll see changes is in the quality of your skin. We often talk about that green smoothie glow. Healthy eating and living will remove years from your face, eliminate wrinkles, fade age spots, and give you a "second youth." Your skin will become supple, and acne will clear up. Your eyes will become brighter and begin to sparkle. The dark circles and puffiness will diminish as will the yellowness in the whites of your eyes. On the inside of your body, your cells will become rejuvenated as well, causing your organs to function more efficiently.

3. *Improved Digestion.* Green smoothies are much easier to digest and metabolize than solid food. Just because you "eat healthy" doesn't mean you are automatically getting all the nutrients necessary for your health and well-being. There are many people whose bodies do not digest solid foods effectively, so the nutrients from the food are not completely absorbed by the body. Green smoothies, which are in a blended, liquid form, are far easier to metabolize. In fact, these delicious smoothies are so bio-available that their nutrients start to get absorbed by the body even while the smoothie is still in your mouth! Processed foods, excessive gluten and proteins, fried foods, and other unhealthy fats are the main reasons behind the digestive issues most of us face. Since green smoothies are thoroughly blended, the majority of the work your digestive system would normally need to do is already done. Your body can then more easily assimilate and extract the nutrients needed for optimum health.

You'll discover other additional health benefits of green smoothies as we go through this book.

SEVEN TIPS FOR GREEN SMOOTHIE SUCCESS

1. *Chew your smoothies.* Yes, chew the liquid smoothie. Try to go through the chewing motion as much as possible, as the saliva in your mouth starts the digestive process. This will also help minimize gas and bloating.

2. *Add protein to your smoothie.* As a nutritionist, I recommend adding 1 to 2 scoops of protein powder to your smoothie because it will help keep you feeling full longer and keep your metabolism revved up. The protein can make the smoothie taste slightly pasty, so try the smoothie first without it and then add the protein to see if it is palatable to you. My favorite type of protein powders are non-dairy, plant-based protein powder, such as rice, soy, or hemp protein.

3. *Keep your smoothies fresh.* It is always ideal to drink your smoothie the same day you blend it to ensure that you get maximum nutrition from it. However, if you are busy or for some other reason can't make them fresh daily, then they can keep extremely well for up to two days in the refrigerator. A glass jar with a lid is ideal

to safely store your smoothies. Covering your green smoothies with a tight lid minimizes oxidation and absorption of other smells from the refrigerator. We're all being pulled in different directions from sunup to sundown, so if preparing them in advance helps you stay on track, I'm all for it.

4. *Rotate your greens each month.* All greens have certain types of alkaloids in them. Now, these alkaloids are in very small, harmless amounts, but if you continually take in the same type of greens week after week, you can get a buildup of that type of alkaloid and suffer serious health consequences. The easiest way to avoid this is to rotate your greens. One week, buy spinach, the next week, kale, the next week, romaine lettuce. Or you can buy two greens for one week and then two different greens the following week. The goal is to rotate different greens into your smoothies each week. There are plenty of green leafy veggies to choose from. When we talk about greens, know that the variety includes spinach, kale, arugula, bok choy, beet greens, Swiss chard, romaine, collards, and dandelion greens.

5. *Make it taste good.* The recipes can be slightly altered to taste. So feel free to add more ice or water if you prefer your smoothies to be thinner. Also, feel free to add more stevia to sweeten, if necessary, or leave the stevia out if your smoothie is sweet enough. Stevia is a natural herbal sweetener that won't cause blood sugar spikes. It's important that the smoothie taste good to you so you will continue with green smoothies.

6. *Don't think diet, think detox.* Although green smoothies are great for weight loss, you don't want to use them as a fad diet. The Green Smoothie Cleanse is meant to detox the body and jump-start weight loss, but it is not a weight-loss plan. Green Smoothies are great to enjoy daily for the nutritional benefits alone. However, fixating on only green smoothies all day, every day for extended periods of time, is unhealthy and could slow our metabolism. Focus on changing your eating habits for life, retraining your taste buds to desire, and crave healthier foods!

7. *Join our Green Smoothie Facebook group.* Get support, encouragement, and tips from me and thousands of others at https://www.facebook.com/groups/Green.Smoothie.Cleanse/.

SEVEN TIPS THAT MENTALLY PREPARE YOU FOR THIS JOURNEY

1. *Make your health a high priority.* You must begin thinking differently. First, decide that your health is one of the top priorities in your life. Know that your body is naturally thin. If you prepare your mind and absorb the knowledge offered to you in this book, you will have all the power you need to become your best self and transform your life in every way. Even if you are a busy mom or a high-powered career executive, know that today begins the journey toward your most amazing, beautiful self. It is time to treat your body as the greatest gift that you have. It is time to shine as the person you were always meant to be. When you have healthy and positive energy in life, amazing things like love, joy, success, and wealth come your way. Every interaction at work, church, home, or in the streets can be simply magnetic. Get healthy, lose weight, and watch your entire life begin to change for the better.

2. *Focus on getting healthy, and the weight loss will follow.* If you're drinking green smoothies for fast weight loss, you're totally missing the point! Getting on the scale every day is a waste of time. You will not lose pounds every day, and guess what, some days you may actually gain weight because your body is adjusting during the weight-loss process. If you focus on fast weight loss, you'll be on a diet for life. Ninety-five percent of people who lose weight on a fad diet gain it back in three to five years. I'm done with dieting! You need to change your eating habits for life. So prepare yourself for the journey. Embrace a lifestyle change where you desire and crave healthy foods, where you never have to count calories and serving sizes, and you truly won't have to diet again. Focus on getting healthy, and the weight loss will follow.

3. *Detox family and friends.* Sometimes you need to detox your emotions as well as your body by withdrawing from family and friends who discourage you, tell you "you can't do it" or "you're not ready to do it." Blah blah blah! If there is negative talk coming from some people in your life, I would encourage you to limit the amount of time you spend with them. We all have enough negative thoughts on our own without people adding to them! Don't gravitate toward people who say you can't do something. Know that when you start this weight-loss journey,

you will want to give up. It's normal. But I know that sometimes the only way to grow in life is to be uncomfortable. How else do you grow mentally, spiritually, and physically? When you cheat or mess up, it's no big deal. You will experience being irritable, doubtful, cranky. And then one day, you will experience the joy, the energy, and the feeling of accomplishment that settles in. Don't you want that feeling?

4. *Understanding the difference between emotional hunger vs. physical hunger.* Sometimes our relationship with food is an emotional one rather than a physical one. Sometimes we eat to fill an emotional gap or some other negative emotion. But no cookie, cracker, cake, ice cream, or pie can satisfy emotional hunger. Emotional hunger comes on suddenly—I must eat something now. But you rarely feel satisfied or full, and so you just keep eating and eating until the entire bag of chips or pint of ice cream is gone. If the hunger comes on after an argument or a negative emotion, then it is emotional hunger. You need to learn to deal with the emotions head-on. Physical hunger comes about gradually every three to four hours. Watch the clock. If you ate a meal and were full one hour ago and then feel a sudden need to eat something, it's probably emotional hunger. Dealing with your emotional issues will help you improve your relationship with food. Just as we can get rid of toxic wastes in the body, we can get rid of toxic emotions as well. Instead of eating to distract ourselves from bad feelings, we need to process and eliminate them—just like the body does with food: it takes the nutrients it needs and expels the rest.

5. *Expect your weight to fluctuate.* On this weight-loss journey, you may gain on some days, while other days you may lose weight. This is perfectly normal. Weight fluctuates due to three things in the body: muscle, fat, and water. Muscle weighs the most—that's why you can work out and build muscle and thereby gain weight. But you're actually making progress by building muscle because it will help you burn fat all day long. For women, water is the biggest culprit, due to our hormones. Many of us gain 5 to 10 pounds of water weight during our cycle. For some, excess salt/sodium causes water to be trapped under the tissues in the body, making us weigh more and look bloated and puffy! So don't panic if your weight

loss is a little up and down. When it's up every week, week after week, *then* you know you have a problem. Also, look into getting a Tanita scale—it will tell you your weight and percentage of muscle, fat, and water in the body. This is helpful for people who work out!

6. *Engage in positive self-talk.* Thoughts and feelings turn into actions, and actions into reality. Remember, you are beginning a new chapter in your life. Let me encourage you right now to get started with your journey. Many ask, "How do I start?" or "How do I get there?" Well, it begins with positive self-talk. You want to stop thinking and saying negative things about yourself. You are not fat, lazy, ugly, or sick. Your true self is naturally thin, beautiful, and healthy. If you have negative thoughts about yourself, you'll attract negative people and outcomes in your life. If you say that you can never lose weight, you're exactly right: you won't. If you say you can, your subconscious mind believes that and begins to move your actions in the direction of losing weight.

7. *Don't get obsessed with weighing yourself every day.* Don't let your bathroom scale ruin your motivation. Frequent weighing can be confusing, so instead focus on how your clothes look and feel on your body. Scales are reliable over the long haul but give you inaccurate day-to-day reads. Weight fluctuations can be caused by hormonal changes or fluid shifts and can lead to unnecessary disappointment. It can show gains or losses that are not there because most basic scales can't tell the difference between fat, muscle, and water weight. Your weight also fluctuates by several pounds throughout the day, and weighing yourself too much will only be confusing and discouraging. Plan on weighing yourself only once a week at the same time of day and wearing the same clothing or no clothing (naked is best). Focus on losing inches and on how you begin to feel, not just on pounds. With this program, you will be doing great things for your body and health. The number on the scale will take care of itself.

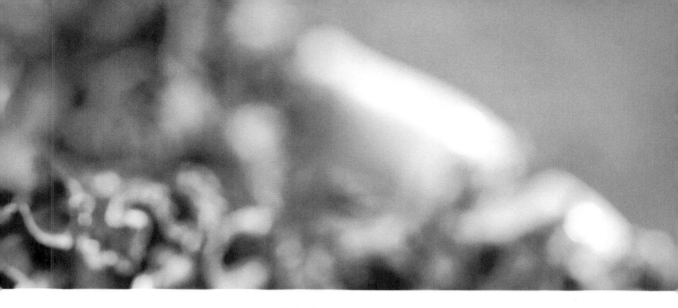

PART 1

30-DAY PROGRAM

This section provides you with the guidelines for completing the 30-Day Program, which consists of a full meal plan for 30 days. You are provided with 30 days of green smoothie recipes, hot meal recipes, snacks, and desserts. It will include the step-by-step prescriptive regimen for you to follow each day, along with shopping lists, recipes, guidelines, and frequently asked questions. All you'll need to do is follow the guidelines for each day and listen to your body. It will reward you for your efforts.

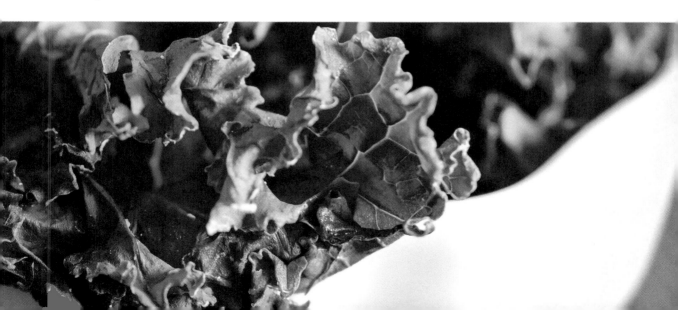

1
How to Do the 30-Day Program

**TO ENSURE SUCCESS ON THE 30-DAY PROGRAM,
FOLLOW THESE SIX SPECIFIC GUIDELINES:**

1. *Drink two green smoothies and eat one healthy meal every day.* Each day, drink one green smoothie for breakfast, one green smoothie for lunch, and eat one healthy meal for dinner. (Note: You can vary this, i.e., drink one for lunch and one for dinner, if you prefer, as long as you drink two per day.) This book provides the green smoothie recipes as well as a healthy meal menu for all 30 days. When you make the green smoothie recipe in the morning, divide it into half, and have half for breakfast and half for lunch. Each green smoothie serving should contain 10 to 14 ounces of liquid. If you take the smoothie out of the house with you to drink it later, keep it refrigerated as much as possible.

2. *Eat snacks to feel full.* The good news for those who already use the 10-Day Green Smoothie Cleanse is that I've expanded the list of snacks. You may snack on apples, popcorn (lightly salted), protein bars, hummus, celery, carrots, cucumbers, broccoli, and other crunchy veggies throughout the day. Other high-protein snacks include unsweetened peanut butter, hard-boiled eggs, and raw or unsalted nuts and seeds (only a handful). Please note that unsweetened peanut butter will have less than 3 grams of sugar.

3. *Enjoy a variety of drinks.* Drink at least eight glasses of water (64 ounces) per day, and drink detox or herbal teas as desired. Ideally, you want to drink the detox tea first thing every morning as it assists in the detox process by cleansing the organs that aid in detoxing—kidneys, liver, and skin. You can also enjoy one cup of coffee or green tea per day. Many experts believe that coffee actually boosts your metabolism so one cup of coffee per day is fine. However, when you need several cups of coffee throughout the day to function, your body is addicted to it and you must break that addiction.

4. *Avoid unhealthy foods.* Do not eat any white sugar, red meat, milk (cow's milk), liquor, beer, sodas/diet sodas, processed foods, fried foods, refined carbs (such as white bread, pastas, and donuts).

5. *Get moving.* It is important to move at least 3 to 5 days per week. You can enjoy any type of physical activity that meets your fitness level, even if it's just walking for 20 to 30 minutes.

6. *Have one optional splurge per week.* You can enjoy a special treat/dessert once a week while on this meal plan. See Chapter 5 Special Treats to find healthy, clean dessert options. To maximize weight loss, it's important to keep desserts to a minimum and not overindulge.

The Menu

DAY	BREAKFAST	LUNCH	DINNER
1	Blueberry Apple Smoothie	Blueberry Apple Smoothie	Cajun Roasted Chicken and Cauliflower
2	Peachy Pineapple Smoothie	Peachy Pineapple Smoothie	Cajun Roasted Chicken and Cauliflower
3	Berry Pineapple Smoothie	Berry Pineapple Smoothie	Salmon Caesar Salad
4	Berry Grape Smoothie	Berry Grape Smoothie	Salmon Caesar Salad
5	Tropical Pineapple Smoothie	Tropical Pineapple Smoothie	Baked Chicken and Veggies
6	Apple Banana Smoothie	Apple Banana Smoothie	Baked Chicken and Veggies
7	Berry Surprise Smoothie	Berry Surprise Smoothie	Spinach Strawberry Salad
8	Blueberry Kale Smoothie	Blueberry Kale Smoothie	Spinach Strawberry Salad
9	Kale Banana Smoothie	Kale Banana Smoothie	Baby Kale Salad with Grilled Scallops
10	Strawberry Banana Smoothie	Strawberry Banana Smoothie	Baby Kale Salad with Grilled Scallops
11	Blueberry Banana Spinach Smoothie	Blueberry Banana Spinach Smoothie	Collards and Black-Eyed Peas
12	Strawberry Pineapple Smoothie	Strawberry Pineapple Smoothie	Collards and Black-Eyed Peas
13	Mixed Berry Banana Smoothie	Mixed Berry Banana Smoothie	Chicken Spinach Salad
14	Blueberry Peach Smoothie	Blueberry Peach Smoothie	Chicken Spinach Salad

DAY	BREAKFAST	LUNCH	DINNER
15	Orange Spinach Smoothie	Orange Spinach Smoothie	Skinny Shrimp Scampi
16	Blueberry Apple Banana Smoothie	Blueberry Apple Banana Smoothie	Skinny Shrimp Scampi
17	Mango Grape Smoothie	Mango Grape Smoothie	Oven-Fried Turkey Cutlets
18	Apple Spring Mix Smoothie	Apple Spring Mix Smoothie	Oven-Fried Turkey Cutlets
19	Mango Banana Smoothie	Mango Banana Smoothie	Italian Shrimp
20	Peachy Banana Smoothie	Peachy Banana Smoothie	Italian Shrimp
21	Blueberry Spinach Smoothie	Blueberry Spinach Smoothie	Sautéed Tomatoes and Spinach
22	Banana Kale Berry Smoothie	Banana Kale Berry Smoothie	Sautéed Tomatoes and Spinach
23	Mango Spinach Smoothie	Mango Spinach Smoothie	Crispy Trout with Lemon and Chickpeas
24	Pineapple Peach Smoothie	Pineapple Peach Smoothie	Crispy Trout with Lemon and Chickpeas
25	Berry Kale Smoothie	Berry Kale Smoothie	Shrimp and Green Beans Salad
26	Strawberry Banana Smoothie	Strawberry Banana Smoothie	Shrimp and Green Beans Salad
27	Blueberry Kale Smoothie	Blueberry Kale Smoothie	Pineapple Peppered Flounder
28	Berry Surprise Smoothie	Berry Surprise Smoothie	Pineapple Peppered Flounder
29	Tropical Pineapple Smoothie	Tropical Pineapple Smoothie	Apple Walnut Spinach Salad
30	Peachy Pineapple Smoothie	Peachy Pineapple Smoothie	Apple Walnut Spinach Salad

Checklist: Monitor Your Progress Daily

DAY	2 GREEN SMOOTHIES	1 HEALTHY MEAL	SNACKS	DRINKS/ WATER	MOVING (PHYSICAL ACTIVITY)
Sample	✓	✓	✓	✓	✓
1					
2					
3					
4					
5					
6					
7					
8					
9					
10					
11					
12					
13					
14					
15					
16					
17					
18					
19					
20					
21					
22					
23					
24					
25					
26					
27					
28					
29					
30					

MAINTAINING YOUR WEIGHT LOSS

HERE ARE A FEW TIPS TO HELP YOU MAINTAIN YOUR WEIGHT LOSS AFTER THE 30 DAYS:

1. *Drink one green smoothie and eat two healthy meals every day.* Never abandon your green smoothies. Each day, drink a green smoothie for breakfast and eat healthy clean meals for lunch and dinner. You can actually replace any meal of the day with one green smoothie, as some enjoy eating a hearty breakfast from time to time, and having their green smoothie for dinner. Drinking a green smoothie will not only help you maintain your weight loss, but feed your body the nutrition it needs as well.

2. *Eat more frequently.* To keep your metabolism revved up, it's important to eat regularly. The goal is to not let more than four hours pass without a meal or snack. We eat every three or four hours because by eating less often you send a signal to your body that it is starving and deprived, causing the body to respond by slowing the metabolic rate and holding on to existing fat reserves in the body. So, eat more. Great snack options are: popcorn, apples, celery, carrots, cucumbers, broccoli, and other crunchy veggies throughout the day. High-protein snacks include unsweetened peanut butter, hard-boiled eggs, low-sodium tuna, and raw or unsalted nuts and seeds (only a handful).

3. *Plan your meals.* When it comes to maintaining weight loss, meal planning is one of the easiest things you can do to ensure your success. The key is to set aside some time each week to do meal planning. Determine which meals you plan to prepare and cook for the entire week. Make one day a week dedicated to grocery shopping and meal planning.

4. *Spend less time in the kitchen.* Making more than one serving for dinner so that there are leftovers for lunch the next day saves a lot of time. Also, you can take your protein (meat) from your dinner and add it to a salad the next day as your lunch. One other tip is to use lettuce wraps with your protein (meat) from dinner to enjoy as your lunch the following day. Boston lettuce works well for wraps. These tips should help save you time and money.

5. *Create a recipe box and a shopping day.* Create a shopping list for your favorite recipes. As you continue to find new dishes you like, you can add them to your recipe box and have them at your fingertips. You can purchase recipe boxes that hold index cards so you can access them quickly and easily. You can also try some of the apps that organize recipes. Identify a day of the week that you will shop and stay consistent with your shopping and meal planning each week.

6. *Enjoy reward meals.* Although maintaining weight loss is a lifelong effort, we can still have some "reward meals" a few times per week. The goal is to keep to your healthy new eating habits and have 2 to 3 "reward meals" throughout the week. I find that as much as I enjoy my reward meals, I begin to look forward to going back to my healthy eating habits because of how they make me look and feel. By adding these reward meals, you also keep your metabolism guessing. This gives you the flexibility to enjoy indulgences and treats as a reward for maintaining a healthy lifestyle long-term.

7. *Get moving and stay active.* It is important to move at least 3 to 5 days per week. You can enjoy any type of physical activity that meets your fitness level, even if it's just walking for 20 to 30 minutes.

8. *Stay accountable.* If you want to maintain your weight loss, you should stay accountable to someone or to a support group, which will help you avoid old habits. To keep motivated, stay active in the support group or join an online forum.

2
Green Smoothie Recipes

Please note that you can switch the greens or fruits in each recipe from time to time, if you prefer. This should not negatively impact results, though you will likely have to change the shopping list. Regarding fruits, it's always best to use frozen fruits, never canned fruits. Also, by design, a few of these recipes duplicate.

DAY 1

BLUEBERRY APPLE

- -

3 handfuls fresh spinach leaves

1½ cups water

2 apples, cored and quartered

2 cups frozen blueberries

2 packets stevia

2 tablespoons ground flaxseeds

Optional: 1 scoop protein powder

Place the spinach and water into the blender and blend until the mixture is a juice-like consistency. Stop the blender and add the apples, blueberries, stevia, flaxseeds, and protein powder (if using). Blend until creamy.

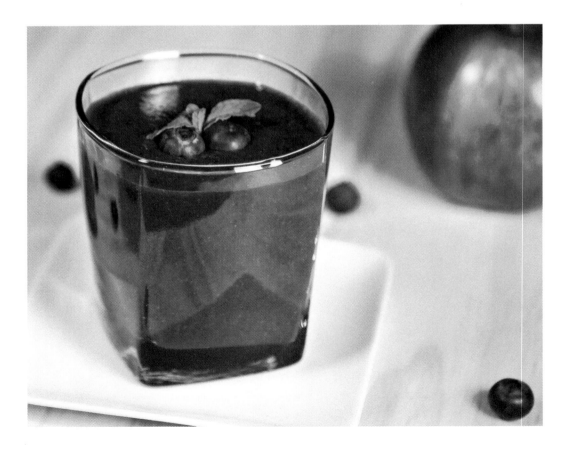

DAY 2

PEACHY PINEAPPLE

- -

3 handfuls fresh spinach leaves

2 cups water

2 cups frozen pineapple chunks

2 cups frozen peach slices

2 packets stevia

2 tablespoons ground flaxseeds

Optional: 1 scoop protein powder

Place the spinach and water into the blender and blend until the mixture is a juice-like consistency. Stop the blender and add the pineapple, peaches, stevia, flaxseeds, and protein powder (if using). Blend until creamy.

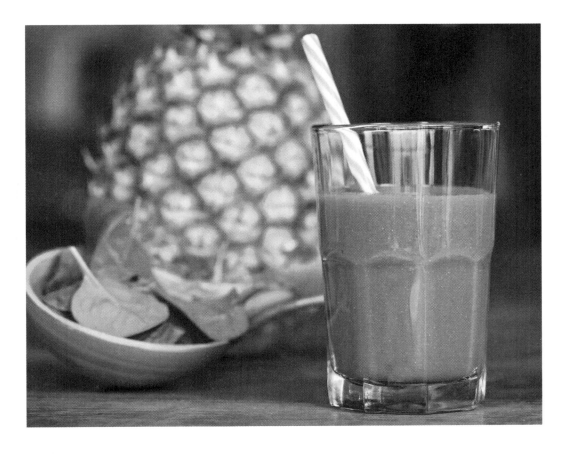

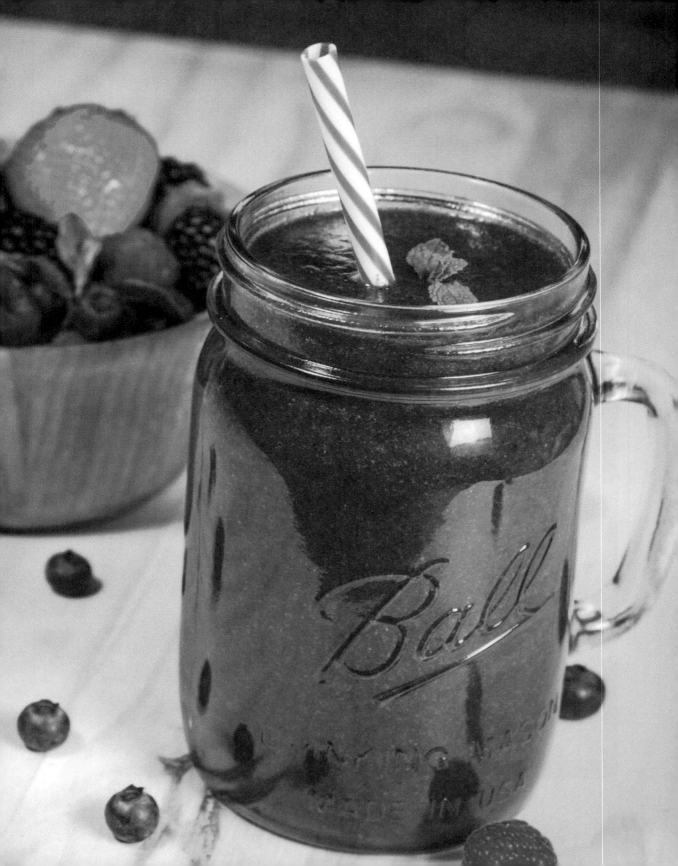

DAY 3

BERRY PINEAPPLE

----

2 handfuls fresh spinach leaves

1 handful fresh kale leaves

2 cups water

2 cups frozen mixed berries

2 cups frozen peach slices

½ cup frozen pineapple chunks

2 packets stevia

2 tablespoons ground flaxseeds

Optional: 1 scoop of protein powder

Place the leafy greens and water into the blender and blend until the mixture is a juice-like consistency. Stop the blender and add the berries, peaches, pineapple, stevia, flaxseeds, and protein powder (if using). Blend until creamy.

DAY 4

BERRY GRAPE

----

3 handfuls fresh spinach leaves

1½ cups water

1 cup fresh or frozen seedless grapes

2 cups frozen blueberries

1 cup frozen pineapple chunks

2 tablespoons ground flaxseeds

Optional: 1 scoop protein powder

Place the spinach and water into the blender and blend until the mixture is a juice-like consistency. Stop the blender and add the grapes, blueberries, pineapple, flax-seeds, and protein powder (if using). Blend until creamy.

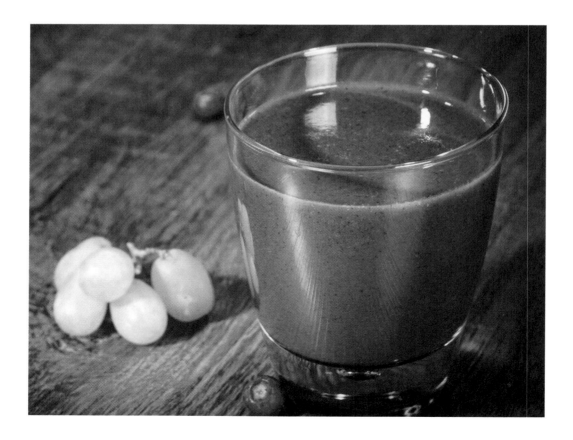

DAY 5

TROPICAL PINEAPPLE

----

3 handfuls fresh spinach leaves

1½ cups water

1 banana, peeled

1 cup frozen peach slices

1 cup frozen pineapple chunks

2 packets stevia

2 tablespoons ground flaxseeds

Optional: 1 scoop protein powder

Place the spinach and water into the blender and blend until the mixture is a juice-like consistency. Stop the blender and add the banana, peaches, pineapple, stevia, flaxseeds, and protein powder (if using). Blend until creamy.

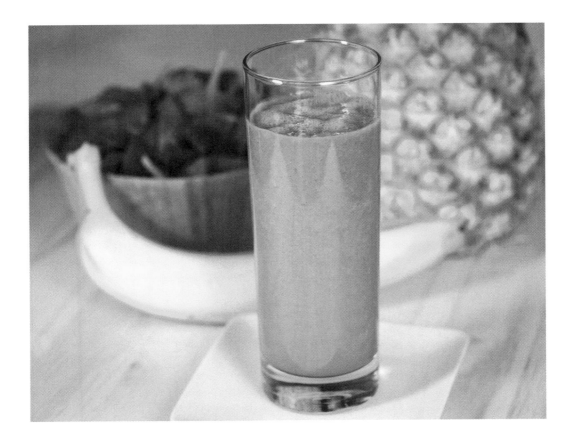

DAY 6

APPLE BANANA

----

3 handfuls fresh spinach leaves

1½ cups water

1 apple, cored and quartered

1 banana, peeled

2 cups frozen blueberries

2 packets stevia

2 tablespoons ground flaxseeds

Optional: 1 scoop protein powder

Place the spinach and water into the blender and blend until the mixture is a juice-like consistency. Stop the blender and add the apple, banana, blueberries, stevia, flaxseeds, and protein powder (if using). Blend until creamy.

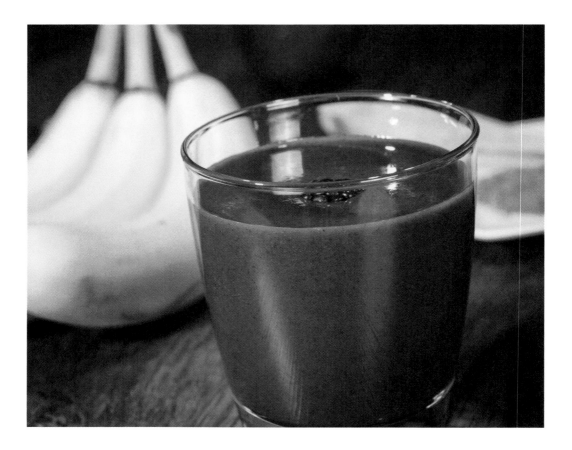

DAY 7

BERRY SURPRISE

- -

3 handfuls fresh spinach leaves

1½ cups water

2 cups frozen pineapple chunks

2 cups frozen mixed berries

2 packets stevia

2 tablespoons ground flaxseeds

Optional: 1 scoop protein powder

Place the spinach and water into the blender and blend until the mixture is a juice-like consistency. Stop the blender and add the pineapple, berries, stevia, flaxseeds, and protein powder (if using). Blend until creamy.

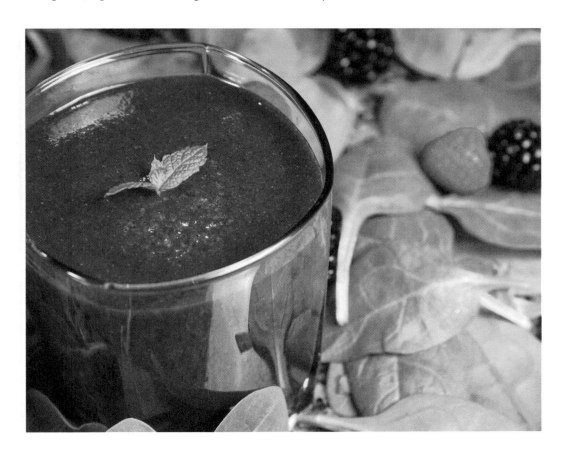

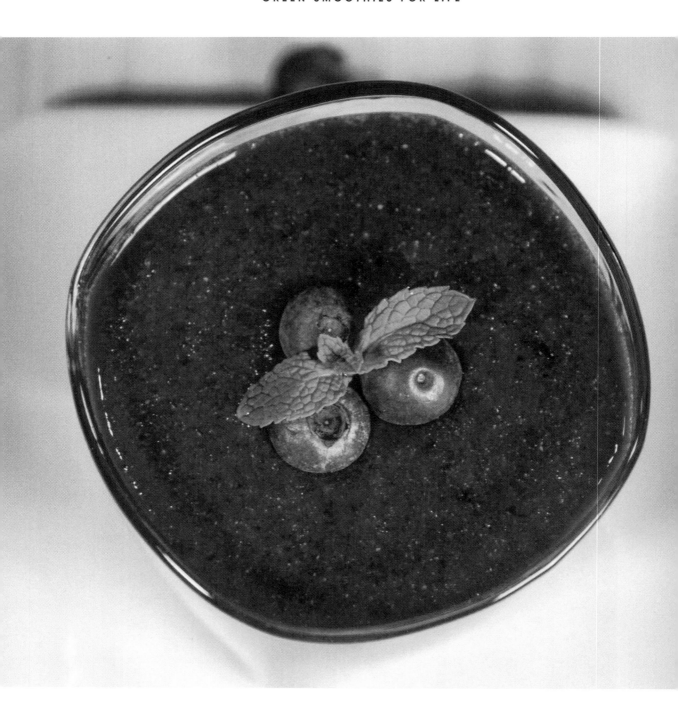

DAY 8

BLUEBERRY KALE

2 handfuls fresh spinach leaves

1 handful fresh kale leaves

1½ cups water

2 cups frozen pineapple chunks

2 cups frozen blueberries

2 packets stevia

2 tablespoons ground flaxseeds

Optional: 1 scoop protein powder

Place the leafy greens and water into the blender and blend until the mixture is a juice-like consistency. Stop the blender and add the pineapple, blueberries, stevia, flaxseeds, and protein powder (if using). Blend until creamy.

DAY 9

KALE BANANA

----

2 handfuls fresh spinach leaves

1 handful fresh kale leaves

1½ cups water

2 cups frozen strawberries

1 cup frozen pineapple chunks

1 banana, peeled

2 packets stevia

2 tablespoons ground flaxseeds

Optional: 1 scoop protein powder

Place the leafy greens and water into the blender and blend until the mixture is a juice-like consistency. Stop the blender and add the strawberries, pineapple, banana, stevia, flaxseeds, and protein powder (if using). Blend until creamy.

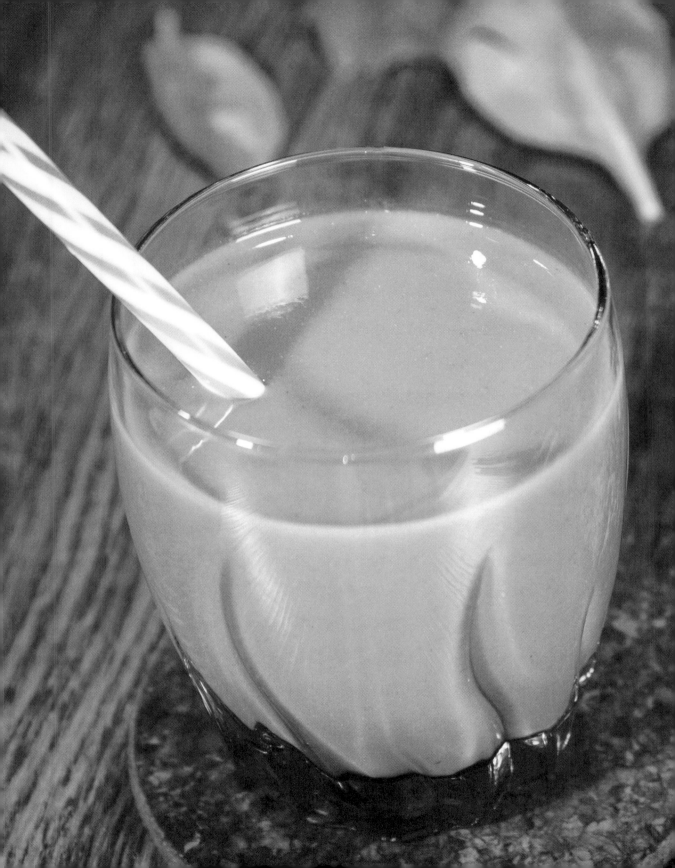

DAY 10

STRAWBERRY BANANA

3 handfuls fresh spinach leaves

1½ cups water

1 cup frozen strawberries

1 banana, peeled

1 cup frozen pineapple chunks

2 packets stevia

2 tablespoons ground flaxseeds

Optional: 1 scoop protein powder

Place the spinach and water into the blender and blend until the mixture is a juice-like consistency. Stop the blender and add the strawberries, banana, pineapple, stevia, flaxseeds, and protein powder (if using). Blend until creamy.

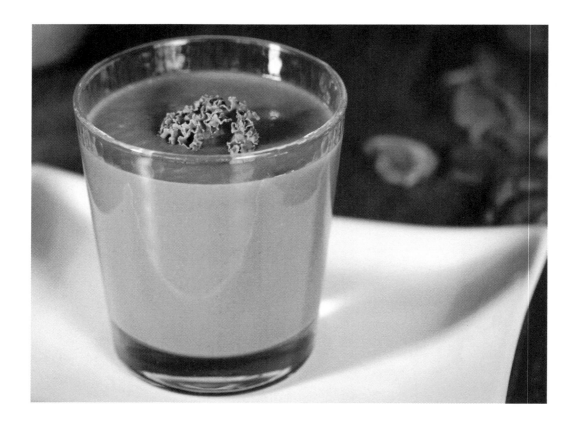

DAY 11

BLUEBERRY BANANA SPINACH

3 handfuls fresh spinach leaves

1½ cups water

1 cup frozen blueberries

1 banana, peeled

2 cups frozen peach slices

2 packets stevia

2 tablespoons ground flaxseeds

Optional: 1 scoop protein powder

Place the spinach and water into the blender and blend until the mixture is a juice-like consistency. Stop the blender and add the blueberries, banana, peaches, stevia, flaxseeds, and protein powder (if using). Blend until creamy.

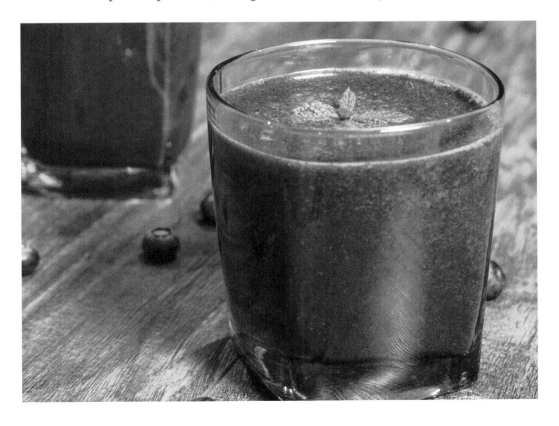

DAY 12
STRAWBERRY PINEAPPLE

----

2 handfuls fresh spinach leaves

1 handful spring mix lettuce leaves

1½ cups water

2 cups frozen pineapple chunks

1 cup frozen strawberries

1 apple, cored and quartered

1 packet stevia

2 tablespoons ground flaxseeds

Optional: 1 scoop protein powder

Place the leafy greens and water into the blender and blend until the mixture is a juice-like consistency. Stop the blender and add the pineapple, strawberries, apple, stevia, flaxseeds, and protein powder (if using). Blend until creamy.

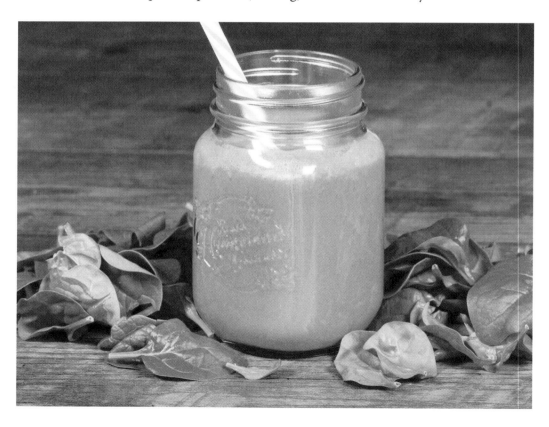

DAY. 13

MIXED BERRY BANANA

3 handfuls fresh spinach leaves

1½ cups water

1 cup frozen mixed berries

1 cup frozen pineapple chunks

1 banana, peeled

1 packet stevia

2 tablespoons ground flaxseeds

Optional: 1 scoop protein powder

Place the spinach and water into the blender and blend until the mixture is a juice-like consistency. Stop the blender and add the berries, pineapple, banana, stevia, flaxseeds, and protein powder (if using). Blend until creamy.

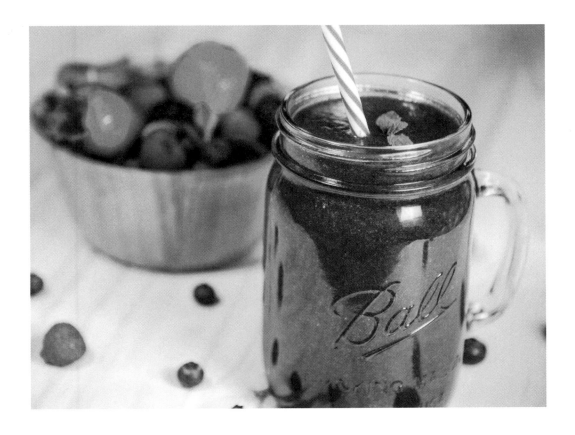

DAY 14

BLUEBERRY PEACH

3 handfuls fresh spinach leaves

1½ cups water

1 cup frozen blueberries

1 cup frozen peach slices

1 cup frozen mango chunks

1 apple, cored and quartered

1 packet stevia

2 tablespoons ground flaxseeds

Optional: 1 scoop protein powder

Place the spinach and water into the blender and blend until the mixture is a juice-like consistency. Stop the blender and add the blueberries, peaches, mango, apple, stevia, flaxseeds, and protein powder (if using). Blend until creamy.

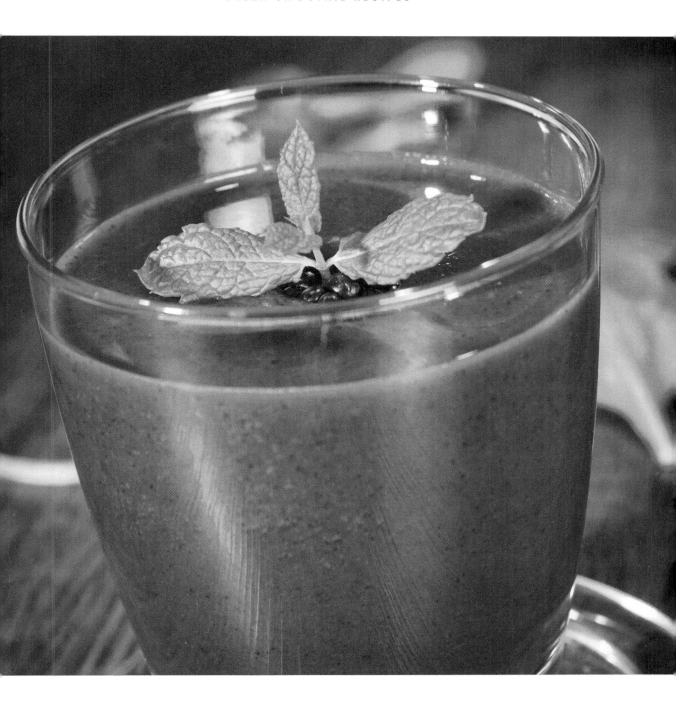

DAY 15

ORANGE SPINACH

3 handfuls fresh spinach leaves

1½ cups water

1 banana, peeled

Juice of 1 orange

1 cup frozen pineapple chunks

1 cup frozen peach slices

1 packet stevia

2 tablespoons ground flaxseeds

Optional: 1 scoop protein powder

Place the spinach and water into the blender and blend until the mixture is a juice-like consistency. Stop the blender and add the orange juice, pineapple, peaches, stevia, flaxseeds, and protein powder (if using). Blend until creamy.

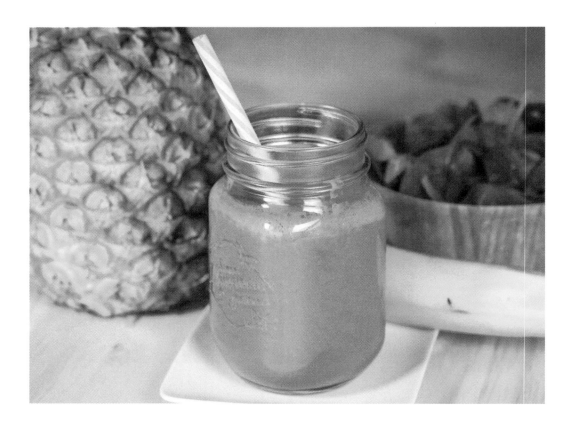

DAY 16

BLUEBERRY APPLE BANANA

3 handfuls fresh spinach leaves

2 cups water

1½ cups frozen blueberries

1 banana, peeled

1 apple, cored and quartered

1 packet stevia

2 tablespoons ground flaxseeds

Optional: 1 scoop protein powder

Place the spinach and water into the blender and blend until the mixture is a juice-like consistency. Stop the blender and add the blueberries, banana, apple, stevia, flaxseeds, and protein powder (if using). Blend until creamy.

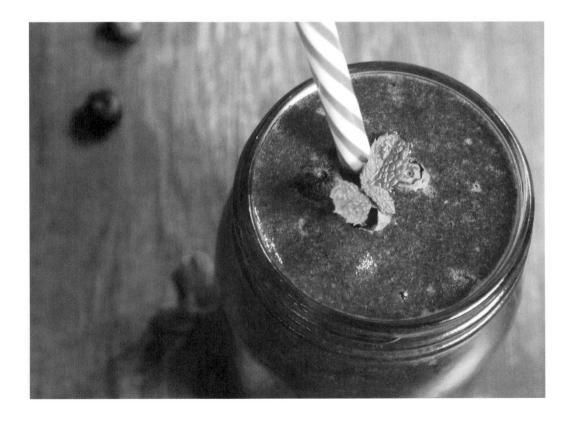

DAY 17

MANGO GRAPE

----

3 handfuls fresh spinach leaves

2 cups water

1 cup frozen mango chunks

1 cup fresh or frozen seedless grapes

1 apple, cored and quartered

1 cup frozen strawberries

1 packet stevia

2 tablespoons ground flaxseeds

Optional: 1 scoop protein powder

Place the spinach and water into the blender and blend until the mixture is a juice-like consistency. Stop the blender and add the mango, grapes, apple, strawberries, stevia, flaxseeds, and protein powder (if using). Blend until creamy.

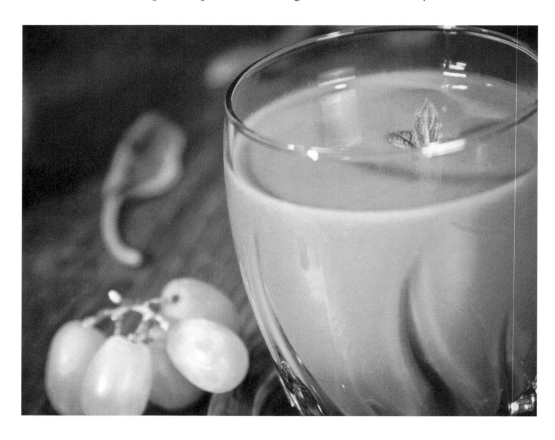

DAY 18

APPLE SPRING MIX

---

2 handfuls spring mix lettuce leaves

1 handful fresh spinach leaves

2 cups water

1 banana, peeled

2 apples, cored and quartered

1½ cups frozen strawberries

2 packets stevia

2 tablespoons ground flaxseeds

Optional: 1 scoop protein powder

Place the leafy greens and water into the blender and blend until the mixture is a juice-like consistency. Stop the blender and add the banana, apples, strawberries, stevia, flaxseeds, and protein powder (if using). Blend until creamy.

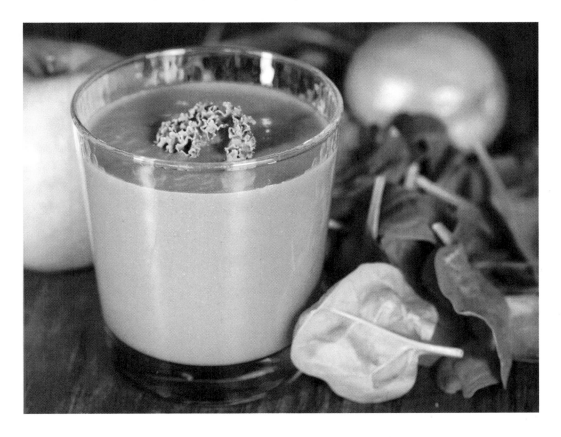

MANGO BANANA

----

2 handfuls spring mix lettuce greens

1 handful fresh spinach leaves

2 cups water

1 banana, peeled

1 cup frozen pineapple chunks

1½ cups frozen mango chunks

1 cup frozen mixed berries

3 packets stevia

2 tablespoons ground flaxseeds

Optional: 1 scoop protein powder

Place the leafy greens and water into the blender and blend until the mixture is a juice-like consistency. Stop the blender and add the banana, pineapple, mango, berries, stevia, flaxseeds, and protein powder (if using). Blend until creamy.

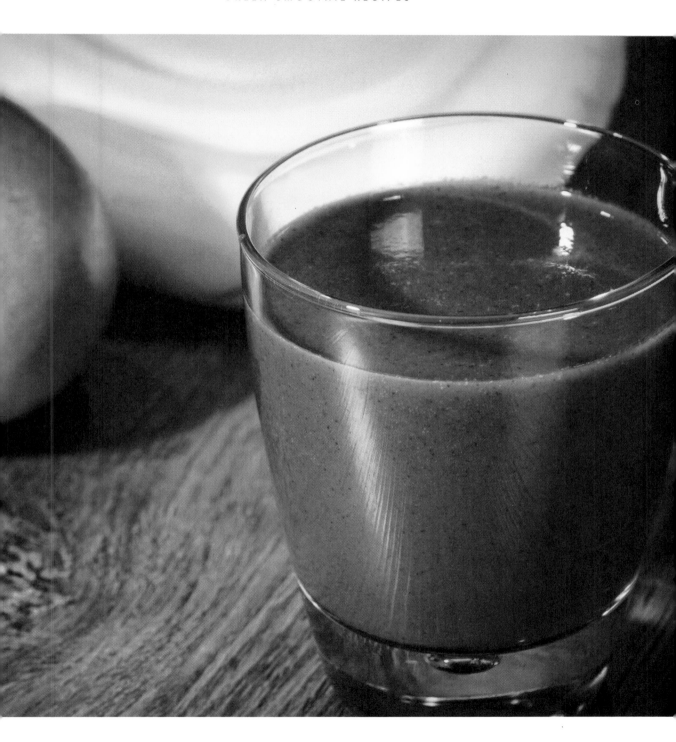

DAY 20

PEACHY BANANA

3 handfuls fresh spinach leaves

2 cups water

1 banana, peeled

1 cup frozen pineapple chunks

2 cups frozen peach slices

1½ packets stevia

2 tablespoons ground flaxseeds

Optional: 1 scoop protein powder

Place the spinach and water into the blender and blend until the mixture is a juice-like consistency. Stop the blender and add the banana, pineapple, peaches, stevia, flaxseeds, protein powder (if using). Blend until creamy.

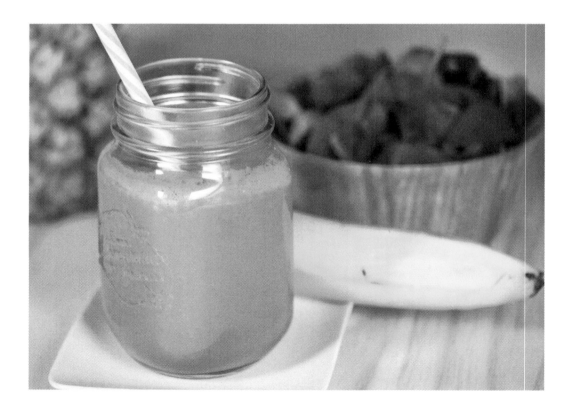

DAY 21

BLUEBERRY SPINACH

----

3 handfuls fresh spinach leaves

2 cups water

1½ cups frozen blueberries

1 cup frozen peach slices

1 cup fresh or frozen seedless grapes

3 packets stevia

2 tablespoons ground flaxseeds

Optional: 1 scoop of protein powder

Place the spinach and water into the blender and blend until the mixture is a juice-like consistency. Stop the blender and add the blueberries, peaches, grapes, stevia, flaxseeds, and protein powder (if using). Blend until creamy.

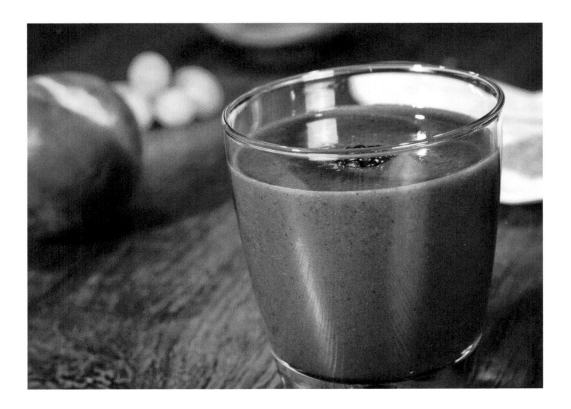

DAY 22

BANANA KALE BERRY

1 handful fresh kale leaves

2 handfuls fresh spinach leaves

2 cups water

2 cups frozen blueberries

1 apple, cored and quartered

1 banana, peeled

2 packets stevia

2 tablespoons ground flaxseeds

Optional: 1 scoop protein powder

Place the leafy greens and water into the blender and blend until the mixture is a juice-like consistency. Stop the blender and add the blueberries, apple, banana, stevia, flaxseeds, and the protein powder (if using). Blend until creamy.

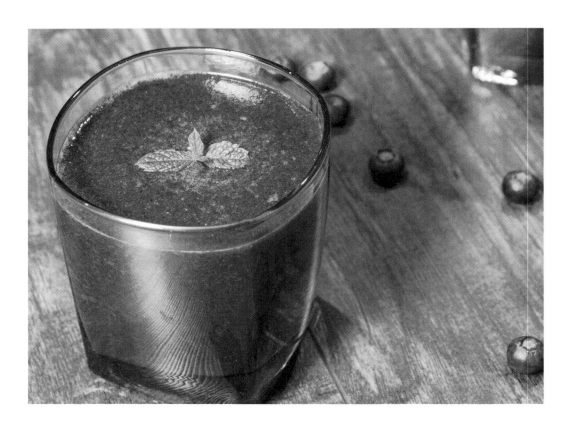

DAY 23

MANGO SPINACH

----

3 handfuls fresh spinach leaves

2 cups water

1 apple, cored and quartered

1½ cups frozen mango chunks

2 cups frozen strawberries

1 packet stevia

2 tablespoons ground flaxseeds

Optional: 1 scoop protein powder

Place the spinach and water into the blender and blend until the mixture is a juice-like consistency. Stop the blender and add the apple, mango, strawberries, stevia, flaxseeds, and protein powder (if using). Blend until creamy.

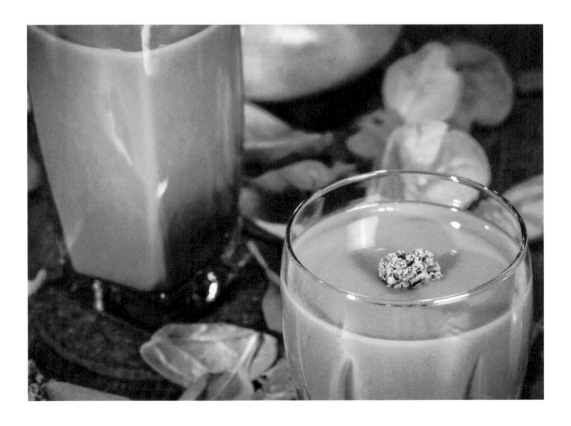

DAY 24

PINEAPPLE PEACH

----

1 handful fresh kale leaves

2 handfuls fresh spinach leaves

2 cups water

1½ cups frozen peach slices

2 cups frozen pineapple chunks

2 packets stevia

2 tablespoons ground flaxseeds

Optional: 1 scoop protein powder

Place the leafy greens and water into the blender and blend until the mixture is a juice-like consistency. Stop the blender and add the peaches, pineapple, stevia, flax-seeds, and protein powder (if using). Blend until creamy.

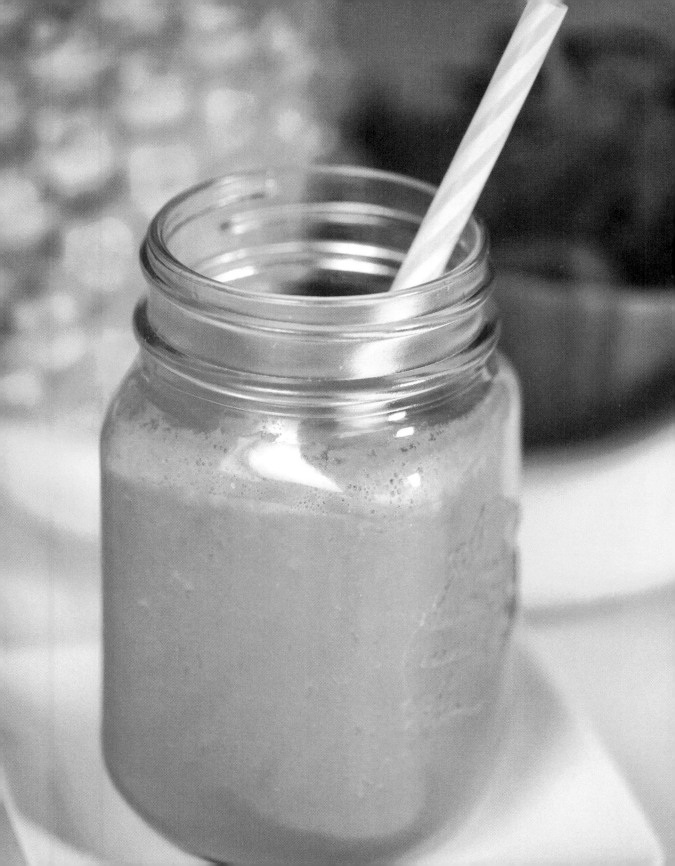

DAY 25

BERRY KALE

----

1 handful fresh kale leaves

2 handfuls fresh spinach leaves

2 cups water

1½ cups frozen mixed berries

1 apple, cored and quartered

1½ cups frozen peach slices

2 packets stevia

2 tablespoons ground flaxseeds

Optional: 1 scoop protein powder

Place the leafy greens and water into the blender and blend until the mixture is a juice-like consistency. Stop the blender and add the berries, apple, peaches, stevia, flaxseeds, protein powder (if using). Blend until creamy.

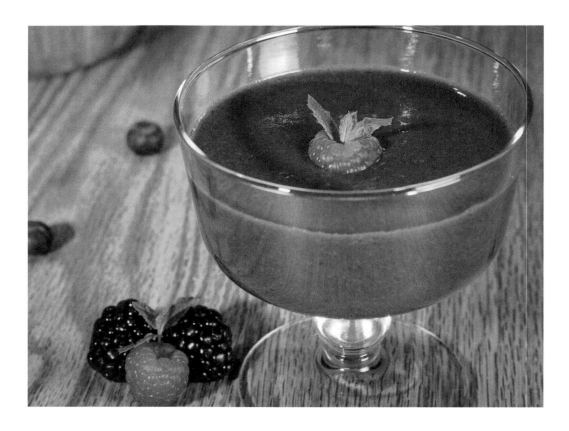

DAY 26

STRAWBERRY BANANA

----

3 handfuls fresh spinach leaves

1½ cups water

1 cup frozen strawberries

1 banana, peeled

1 cup frozen pineapple chunks

2 packets stevia

2 tablespoons ground flaxseeds

Optional: 1 scoop protein powder

Place the spinach and water into the blender and blend until the mixture is a juice-like consistency. Stop the blender and add the strawberries, banana, pineapple, stevia, flaxseeds, and protein powder (if using). Blend until creamy.

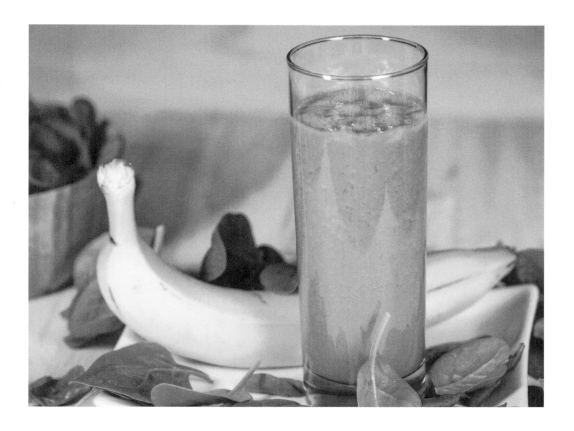

DAY 27

BLUEBERRY KALE

----

1 handful fresh kale leaves

2 handfuls fresh spinach leaves

1½ cups water

2 cups frozen pineapple chunks

2 cups frozen blueberries

2 packets stevia

2 tablespoons ground flaxseeds

Optional: 1 scoop protein powder

Place the leafy greens and water into the blender and blend until the mixture is a juice-like consistency. Stop the blender and add the pineapple, blueberries, stevia, flaxseeds, and protein powder (if using). Blend until creamy.

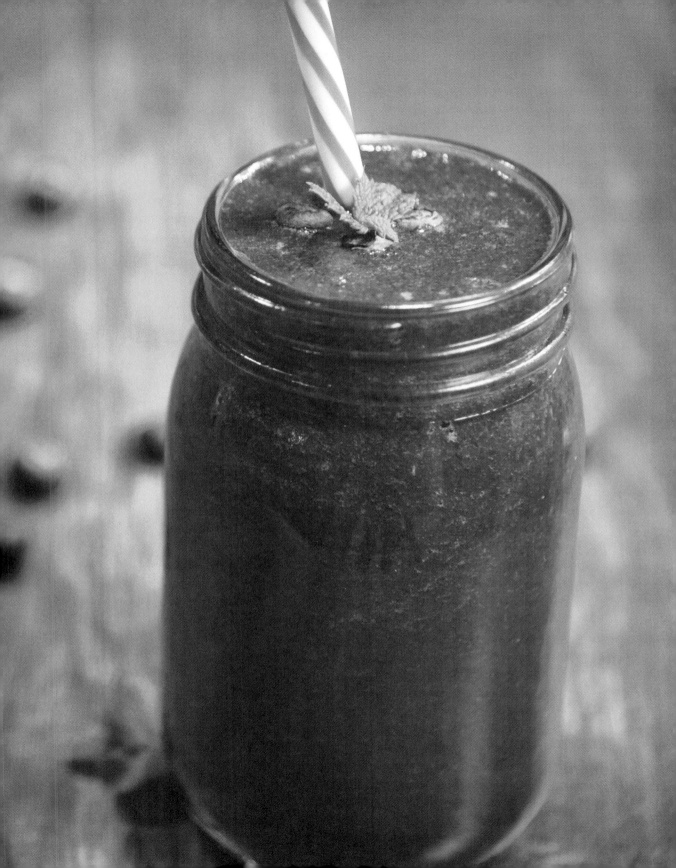

DAY 28

BERRY SURPRISE

----

3 handfuls fresh spinach leaves

1½ cups water

2 cups frozen pineapple chunks

2 cups frozen mixed berries

2 packets stevia

2 tablespoons ground flaxseeds

Optional: 1 scoop protein powder

Place the spinach and water into the blender and blend until the mixture is a juice-like consistency. Stop the blender and add the pineapple, berries, stevia, flaxseeds, and protein powder (if using). Blend until creamy.

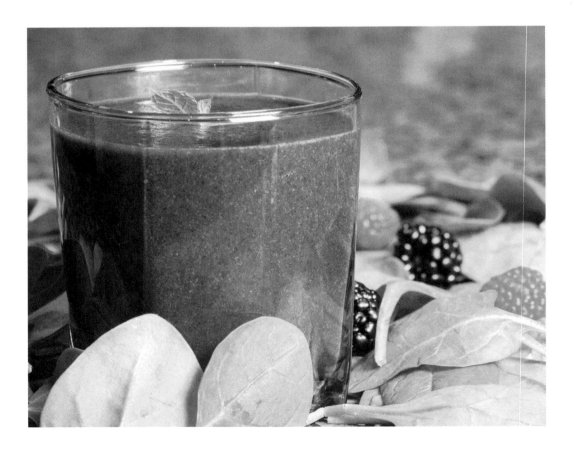

DAY 29

TROPICAL PINEAPPLE

----

3 handfuls fresh spinach leaves

1½ cups water

1 banana, peeled

1 cup frozen peach slices

1 cup frozen pineapple chunks

2 packets stevia

2 tablespoons ground flaxseeds

Optional: 1 scoop protein powder

Place the spinach and water into the blender and blend until the mixture is a juice-like consistency. Stop the blender and add the banana, peaches, pineapple, stevia, flaxseeds, and protein powder (if using). Blend until creamy.

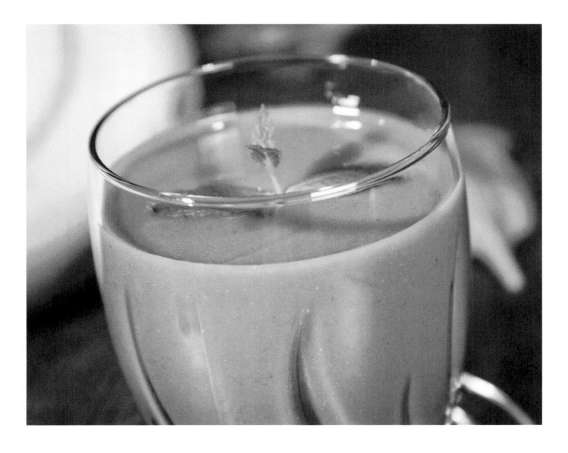

DAY 30

PEACHY PINEAPPLE

----

3 handfuls fresh spinach leaves

2 cups water

2 cups frozen pineapple chunks

2 cups frozen peach slices

2 packets stevia

2 tablespoons ground flaxseeds

Optional: 1 scoop protein powder

Place the spinach and water into the blender and blend until the mixture is a juice-like consistency. Stop the blender and add the pineapple, peaches, stevia, flaxseeds, and protein powder (if using). Blend until creamy.

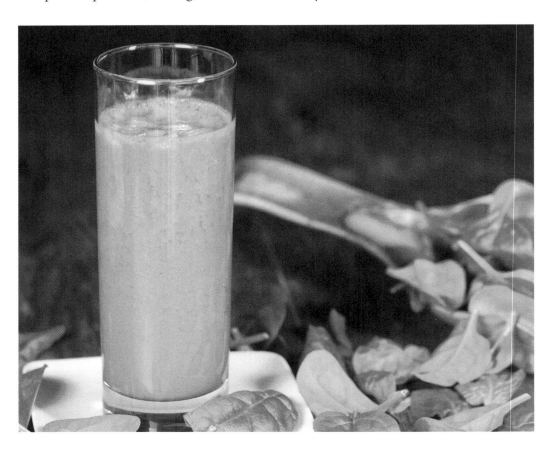

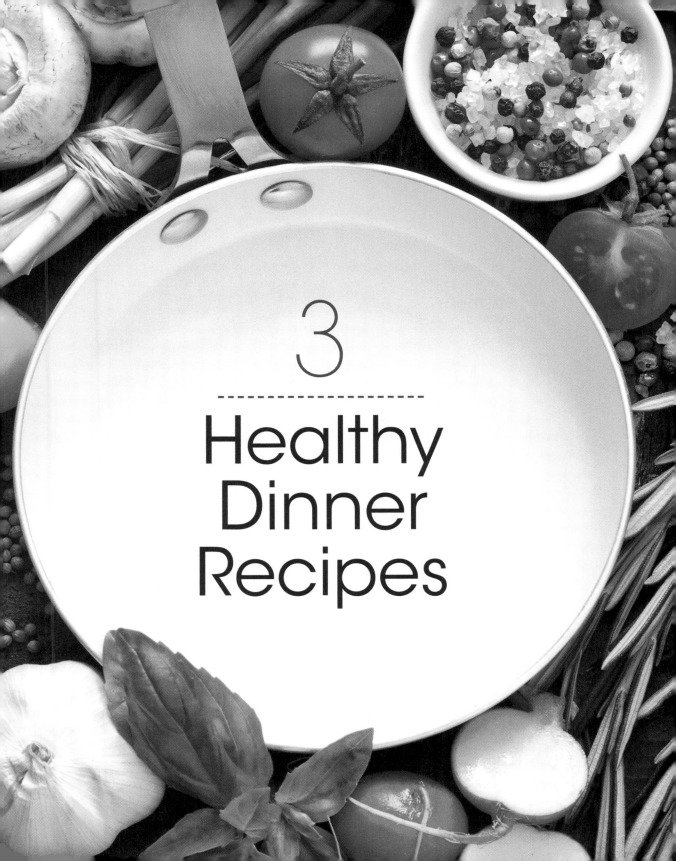

3

Healthy Dinner Recipes

DAYS 1 & 2

CAJUN ROASTED CHICKEN AND CAULIFLOWER

----

2 SERVINGS

1 pound boneless, skinless chicken breasts, cut into ½-inch-wide strips

1 small cauliflower head, trimmed and separated into small florets

1 medium red bell pepper, stemmed, seeded, and cut into thin strips

1 medium yellow bell pepper, stemmed, seeded, and cut into thin strips

3 tablespoons extra-virgin olive oil

1 tablespoon dry Cajun seasoning blend

2 tablespoons red wine vinegar

Preheat the oven to 375°F.

Toss the chicken, cauliflower, and red and yellow bell peppers with the oil and Cajun seasoning until evenly coated in a large roasting pan.

Put the pan in the oven and roast for 25 minutes, stirring a few times, or until the chicken is cooked through and the vegetables are tender.

Remove from the oven and sprinkle the vinegar over the chicken. Before serving, scrape up any browned bits in the pan and add to the final dish.

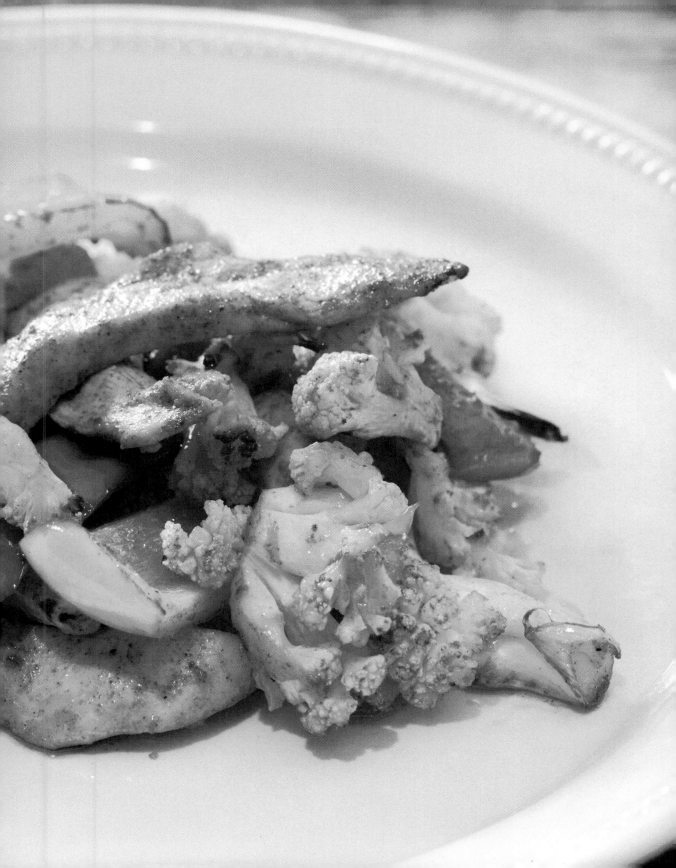

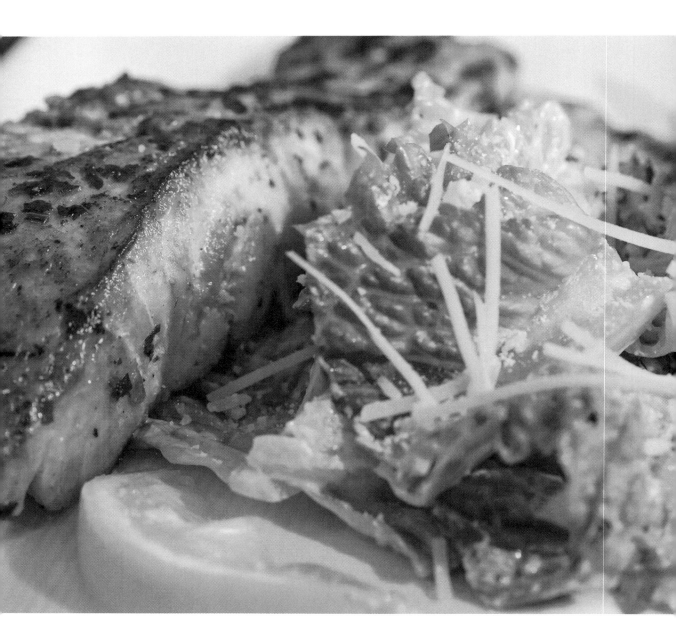

DAYS 3 & 4

SALMON CAESAR SALAD

----

2 SERVINGS

1 teaspoon garlic salt

½ teaspoon lemon pepper

2 (5- to 6-ounce) salmon fillets, skin removed

1 tablespoon extra-virgin olive oil

2 romaine lettuce hearts, rinsed and patted dry

½ cup Caesar dressing (low-sodium)

1 tablespoon Parmesan cheese, grated

Freshly ground black pepper to taste

Sprinkle garlic salt and lemon pepper on the salmon.

Heat a sauté pan over medium-high heat, add the oil, and swirl to coat the pan.

Add the salmon and cook for 2 to 3 minutes until underside is evenly browned and slightly crisp.

Turn the salmon and cook for 4 to 6 minutes or until it reaches the desired temperature.

While the salmon is cooking, tear the romaine into bite-size pieces and place in a large bowl.

Add the dressing, Parmesan, and black pepper. Toss until all the ingredients are well combined.

Cut each salmon fillet in half, place on top of the salad, and serve.

DAYS 5 & 6

BAKED CHICKEN
AND VEGGIES

----

2 SERVINGS

2 pounds chicken, quartered
and skin removed

Sea salt

Freshly ground black pepper

1 lemon, halved

3 tablespoons extra-virgin
olive oil

1 cup broccoli florets

1 cup chopped baby carrots, cut
into ½-inch pieces

1 small red onion, thinly sliced

2 tablespoons chopped
fresh dill

Preheat the oven to 500°F.

Rinse the chicken and pat dry.

Season with the salt and pepper, and place in a roasting pan.

Squeeze ½ of the lemon over the chicken and drizzle with 1 tablespoon of the oil.

Place the chicken in the oven and roast for 15 minutes.

Toss the broccoli, carrots, and onion with the remaining 2 tablespoons oil in a
bowl and season with salt and pepper.

Remove the chicken from oven and scatter the vegetables around it.

Return the pan to the oven and roast for 20 to 25 minutes, until the vegetables
are tender and the chicken is golden and cooked through.

Remove the chicken from the oven and squeeze the remaining ½ lemon over the
chicken and vegetables.

Top with the dill and season with salt and pepper before serving.

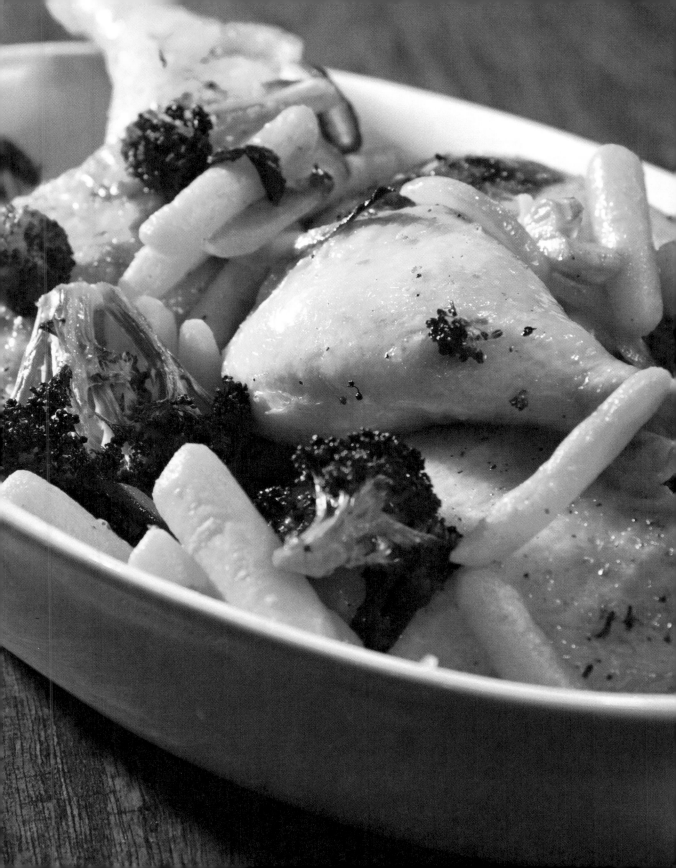

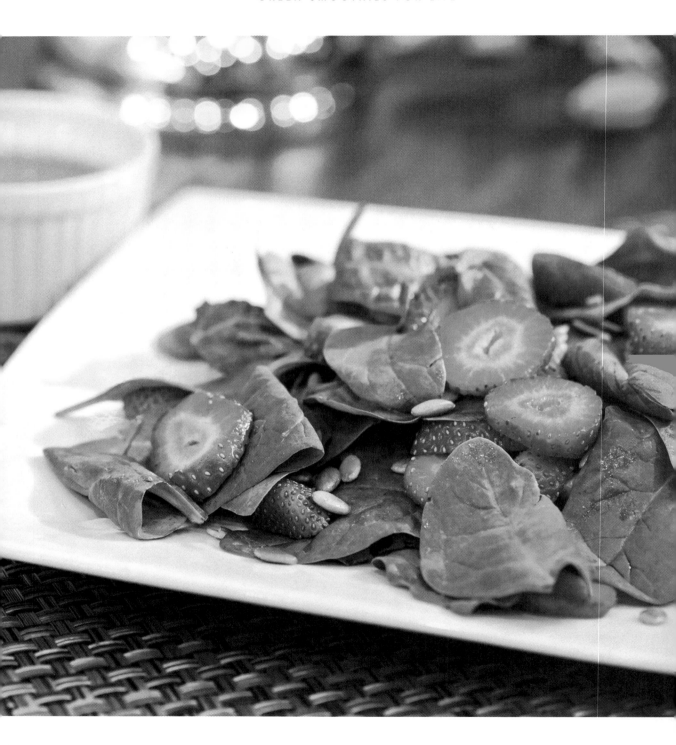

DAYS 7 & 8

SPINACH STRAWBERRY SALAD

----

2 SERVINGS

5 cups loosely packed baby spinach

1 cup strawberries, washed, hulled, and sliced

¼ cup pumpkin seeds, toasted

VINAIGRETTE

¼ cup extra-virgin olive oil

2 tablespoons red wine vinegar

1 teaspoon Dijon mustard

1 teaspoon agave

Pinch of sea salt

Place the spinach and ½ cup of the strawberries in a large bowl.

Make the vinaigrette: In a small bowl, whisk together the oil, vinegar, mustard, agave, and salt.

Pour the vinaigrette over the spinach and strawberry salad and toss to coat evenly.

Top with the pumpkin seeds and the remaining ½ cup strawberries. Serve in bowls.

DAYS 9 & 10

BABY KALE SALAD WITH GRILLED SCALLOPS

----

2 SERVINGS

1½ cups canned black beans, drained and rinsed

2 roasted red peppers (from a jar), drained and chopped

2 tablespoons juice from the red pepper jar

2 tablespoons balsamic vinegar

2 tablespoons extra-virgin olive oil

6 cups packed baby kale leaves

1 tablespoon coconut oil

1 pound sea scallops

½ teaspoon salt

½ teaspoon freshly ground black pepper

Mix the beans, red peppers, red pepper juice, vinegar, and olive oil in a large serving bowl until well combined. Set aside.

Place the baby kale on top of the dressing in the bowl. Do not toss.

Melt the coconut oil in a large skillet over medium heat.

Season the scallops with salt and pepper. Place them in the skillet and cook for 4 minutes, turning once, until browned and cooked through.

Toss the salad in the bowl. Divide it between the serving plates. Set the scallops on top of the salad on each plate and serve.

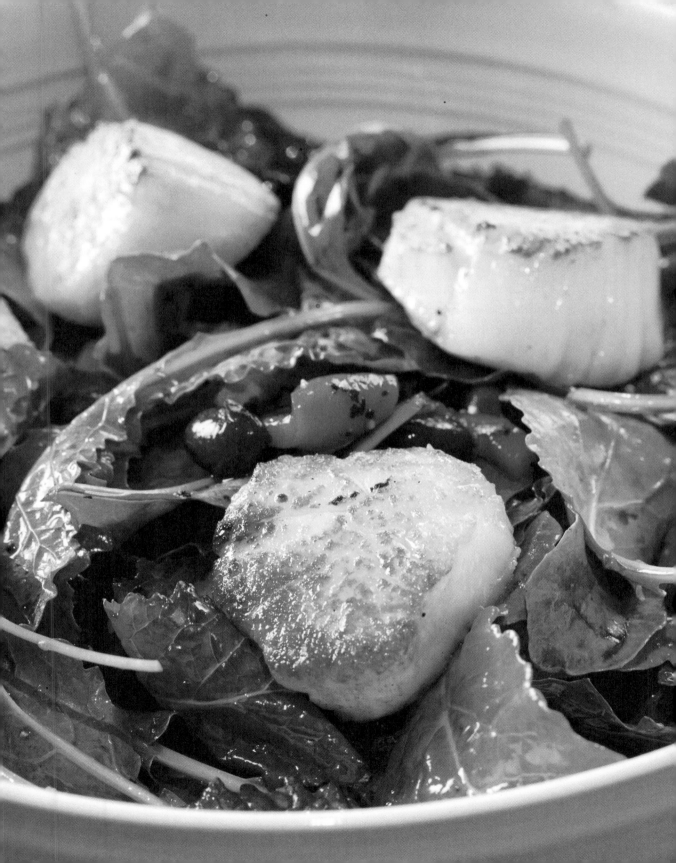

DAYS 11 & 12

COLLARDS AND BLACK-EYED PEAS

----

2 SERVINGS

3 pounds collard greens, washed

4 tablespoons extra-virgin olive oil

4 garlic cloves, minced

1 red onion, diced

3 cups black-eyed peas, rinsed and drained

Dash of apple cider vinegar

Sea salt

Freshly ground black pepper

Chop the collard greens into bite-size pieces.

Heat the oil over medium heat in a large pot and sauté the garlic and onion until soft.

Add the collard greens and stir until wilted; add extra water as needed to prevent the collards from burning.

Add the black-eyed peas and vinegar, and continue cooking for 5 to 6 minutes, until the dish is heated throughout. Season to taste with sea salt and pepper and serve.

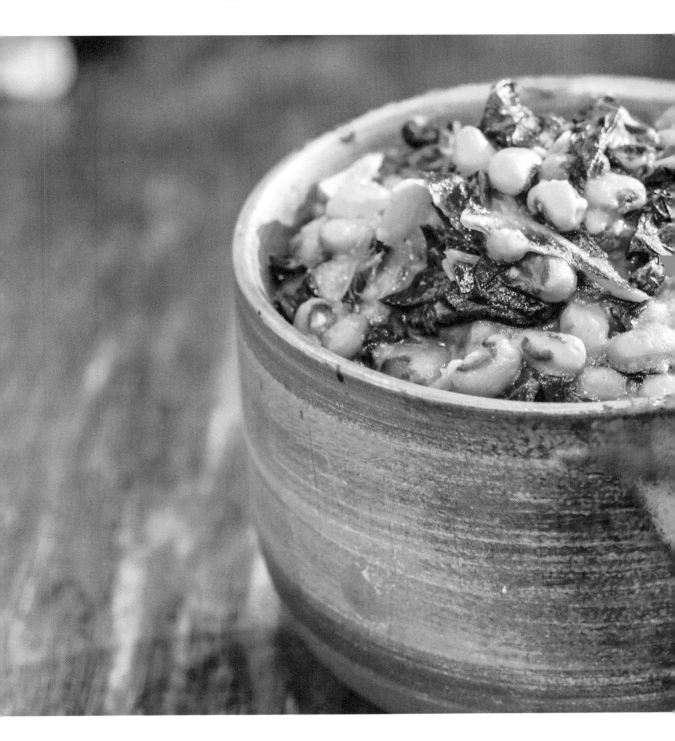

DAYS 13 & 14

CHICKEN SPINACH SALAD

2 SERVINGS

DRESSING

2 tablespoons red wine vinegar

1 teaspoon Dijon mustard

¾ teaspoon salt

¼ teaspoon freshly ground black pepper

⅓ cup extra-virgin olive oil

⅔ pound boneless grilled chicken breast, diced (store-cooked is fine)

1 pound baby spinach (about 8 cups) rinsed and patted dry

¾ cup chopped walnuts

1 small red onion, diced

1 apple, peeled, cored, and cut into small pieces

Make the dressing: In a small bowl, whisk the vinegar with the mustard, salt, and pepper. Whisk in the oil.

Combine the chicken with 2 tablespoons of the dressing in a large bowl.

Let the chicken sit for about 15 minutes to absorb the flavors.

Toss in the spinach, walnuts, onion, apple, and the remaining dressing. Mix until evenly combined.

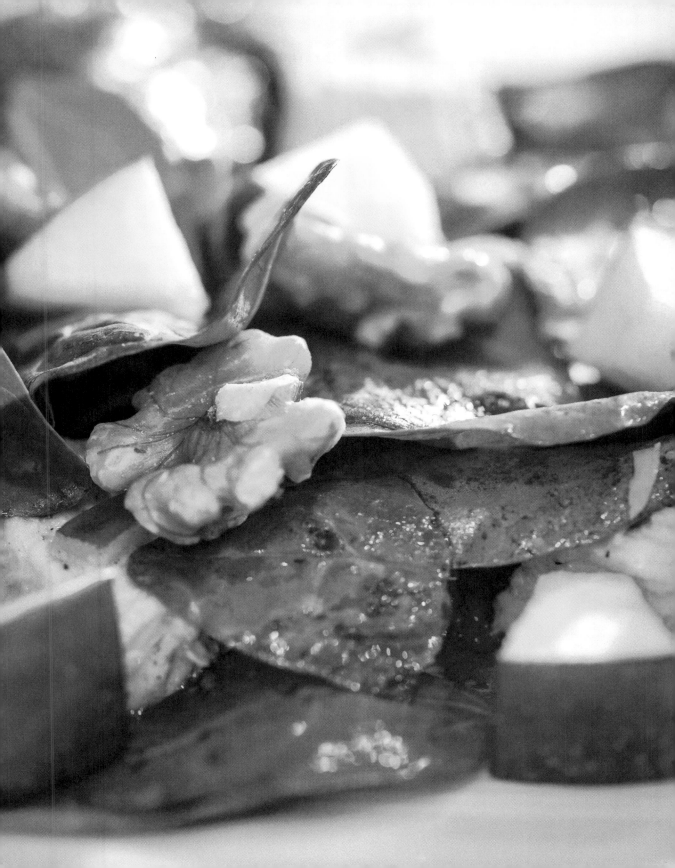

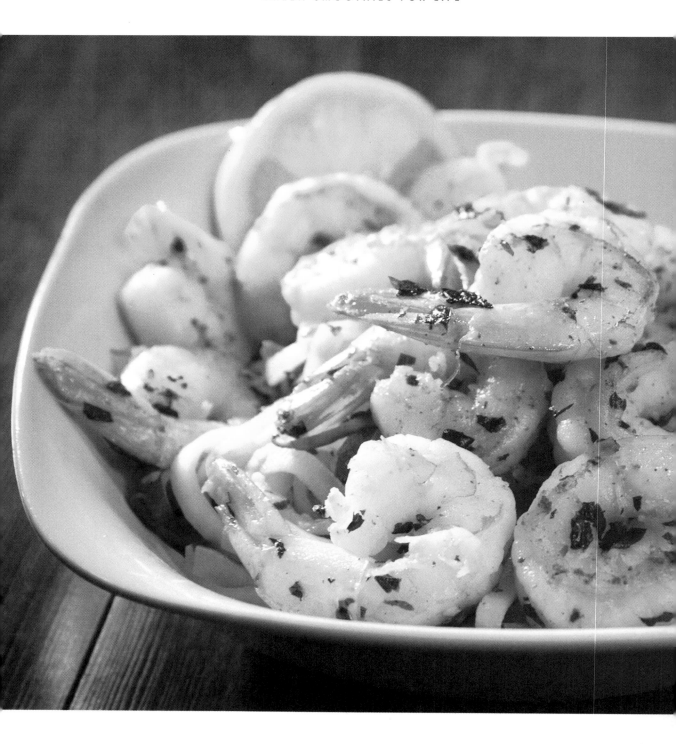

DAYS 15 & 16

SKINNY SHRIMP SCAMPI

----

2 SERVINGS

2 tablespoons extra-virgin olive oil

1 tablespoon minced garlic

¼ teaspoon crushed red pepper flakes

1 pound jumbo shrimp, shelled and deveined

Salt

Freshly ground black pepper

¼ cup dry white wine

2 tablespoons fresh lemon juice

3 small zucchini, or 2 large, cut into noodles

Place a large sauté pan over medium-low heat.

Add the oil and heat for 1 minute. Add the garlic and red pepper flakes, and cook for 1 minute, stirring constantly.

Add the shrimp, stirring as needed, until cooked throughout and pink on all sides, about 3 minutes.

Season the shrimp with salt and pepper and transfer it to a bowl, leaving the liquid in the pan.

Increase the heat to medium. Add the wine and lemon juice to the pan and cook for 2 minutes.

Add the zucchini noodles and cook, stirring occasionally, for 2 to 3 minutes.

Return the shrimp to pan and toss to combine.

Season with salt and pepper and serve immediately.

OVEN-FRIED TURKEY CUTLETS

----

4 SERVINGS

Coconut oil spray

¼ cup ground pecans

¼ cup minced fresh parsley

2 tablespoons grated Parmesan cheese

1 teaspoon finely grated lemon zest

½ teaspoon grated nutmeg

½ teaspoon salt

½ teaspoon freshly ground black pepper

4 (4-ounce) turkey cutlets

Preheat the oven to 375°F.

Lightly coat a large baking sheet with coconut oil spray.

Stir the pecans, parsley, Parmesan, lemon zest, nutmeg, salt, and pepper on a large plate.

Dredge the cutlets in the pecan mixture, coating both sides.

Place the cutlets on the baking sheet and spray the top of each cutlet with coconut oil spray.

Bake for 20 minutes, or until the cutlets are golden brown, particularly at the edges.

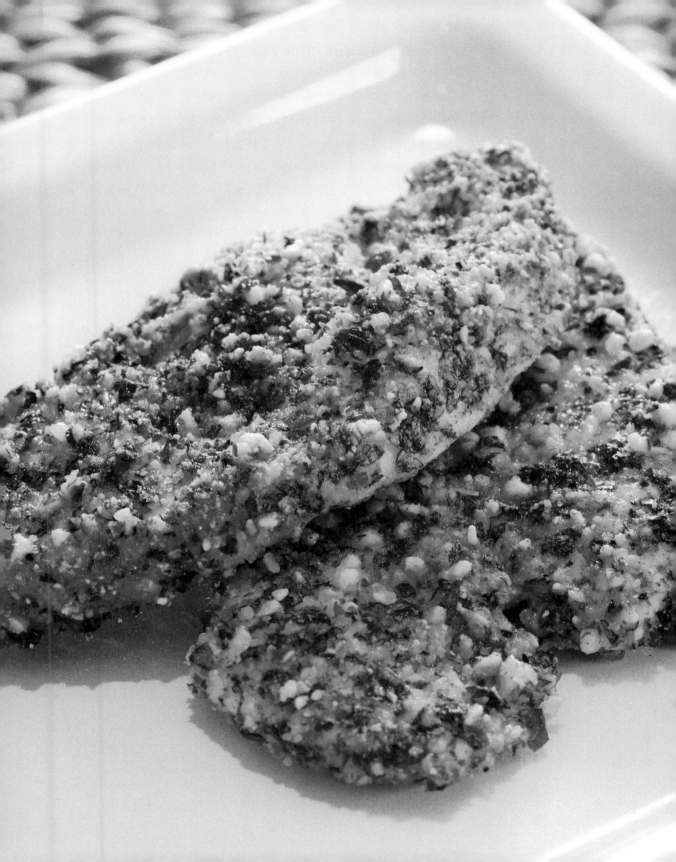

ITALIAN SHRIMP

----

2 SERVINGS

1 pound fresh precooked shrimp

1 teaspoon garlic powder

1 tablespoon dried basil

2 tablespoons tomato paste (no added sugar)

1 tablespoon extra-virgin olive oil

Juice of ½ lemon

Salt

Freshly ground black pepper

Heat the oil in a sauté pan over medium heat and add the shrimp, garlic powder, basil, and tomato paste. Stir to combine and cook, stirring until the shrimp are warmed through.

Squeeze the lemon juice over the shrimp, add salt and pepper to taste, and serve.

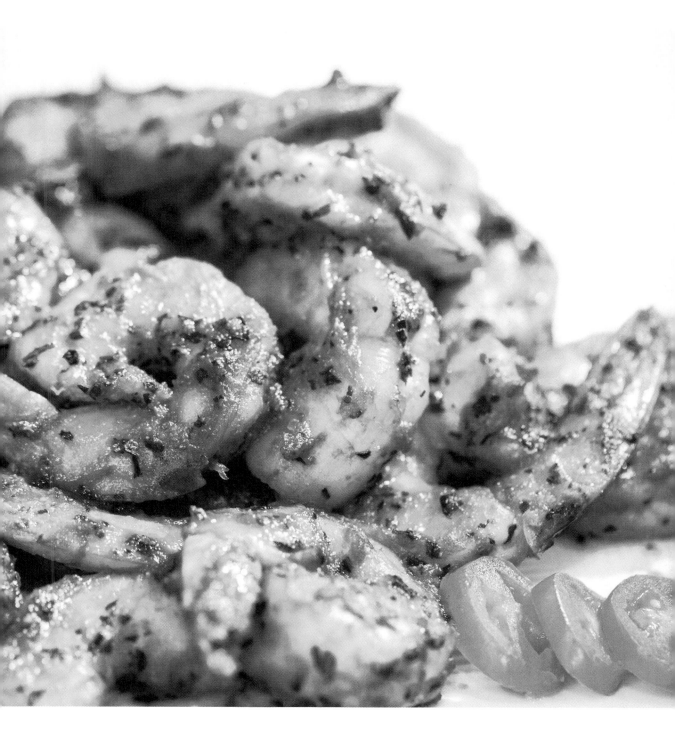

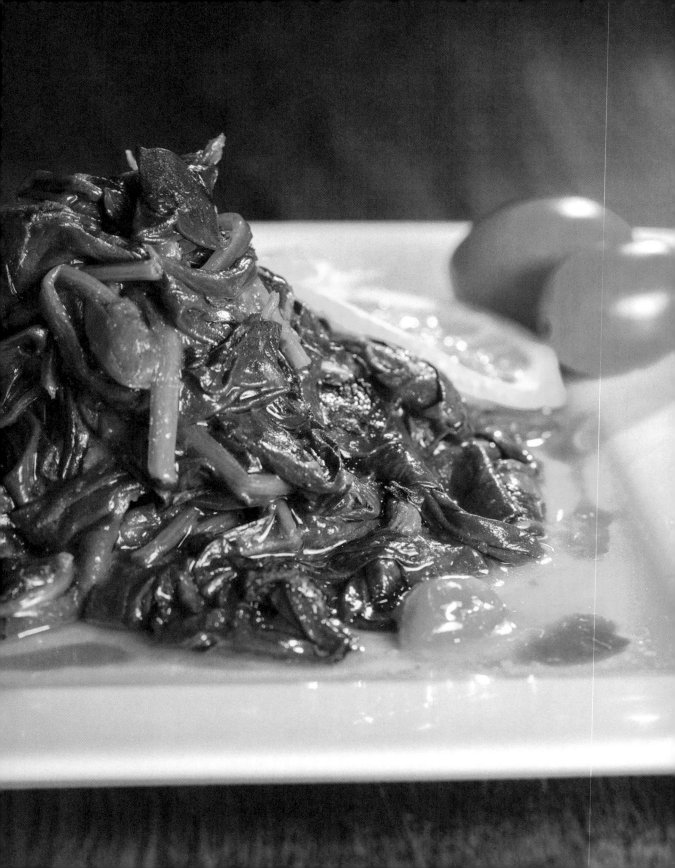

DAYS 21 & 22

SAUTÉED TOMATOES AND SPINACH

----

2 SERVINGS

4 tablespoons grapeseed oil

2 small red onions, finely chopped

4 teaspoons grated fresh ginger

5 small garlic cloves, minced

1 teaspoon sea salt

4 plum tomatoes, seeded and diced

6 cups baby spinach

1 lemon

Heat a large skillet over medium-high heat, add the oil and onions, and sauté for 2 minutes.

Add the ginger, garlic, and salt, and sauté for 30 to 45 seconds. Add the tomatoes and sauté for about 2 minutes.

Add the spinach and cook until wilted, adding splashes of water to prevent the spinach from sticking to the skillet and burning. Season with salt and lemon, and serve.

CRISPY TROUT WITH LEMON AND CHICKPEAS

----

2 SERVINGS

½ teaspoon ground cumin

½ teaspoon salt

½ teaspoon freshly ground black pepper

2 (8-ounce) trout fillets, each halved across the middle

3 tablespoons extra-virgin olive oil

2 large shallots, cut into half-moon rings

1 cup canned chickpeas, rinsed and drained

1 teaspoon minced garlic

1 teaspoon fresh thyme, stems removed

1½ tablespoons lemon juice

Mix the cumin, salt, and pepper in a small bowl. Sprinkle the mixture over the fillets.

Heat 2 tablespoons of the oil in a large skillet over medium heat.

Add the fillets and cook, turning once, for 7 minutes, or until cooked through. Transfer to serving plates.

Pour the remaining 1 tablespoon oil into the skillet. Add the shallots and cook, stirring often, for 2 minutes, or until softened.

Stir in the chickpeas, garlic, and thyme, and cook for 1 minute, stirring constantly.

Add the lemon juice, stir well, and spoon the shallot sauce over the fillets to serve.

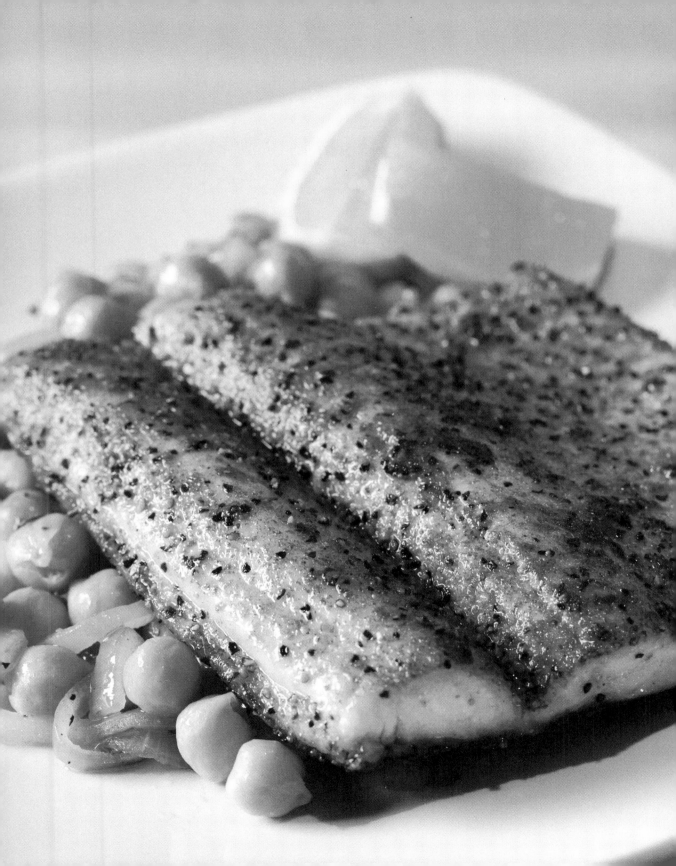

DAYS 25 & 26

SHRIMP AND GREEN BEAN SALAD

2 SERVINGS

MARINADE

4 large garlic cloves, peeled

¼ cup extra-virgin olive oil

2 tablespoons key lime juice

1 teaspoon dried rosemary

½ teaspoon garlic salt

1 pound large shrimp, peeled and deveined

1 pound fresh green beans, trimmed

¼ cup of extra-virgin olive oil

1 teaspoon minced garlic

½ red onion, thinly sliced

Salt

½ teaspoon freshly ground black pepper

½ cup crumbled feta cheese

Make the marinade: Place the garlic cloves, oil, key lime juice, rosemary, and garlic salt in a blender and puree until smooth.

Pour the marinade in a resealable plastic bag and add the shrimp. Marinate for at least 30 minutes in the refrigerator.

Preheat the oven to the broiler setting and place the oven rack on the highest level.

Line a baking sheet with aluminum foil. Pour the shrimp and marinade onto the baking sheet. Place the shrimp in the oven and broil for 3 to 4 minutes per side. Once fully cooked, transfer the shrimp to a bowl.

Bring a large pot of lightly salted water to a boil. Add the green beans and cook for 4 to 5 minutes, until tender. Drain and place the beans in a large bowl.

Heat the oil in a large pan over medium heat. Stir in the minced garlic and the onion, and cook until the onion has softened.

Pour the garlic-onion mixture over the beans, add the shrimp, and toss. Season with salt and pepper, and mix well.

Mix in the feta and serve immediately.

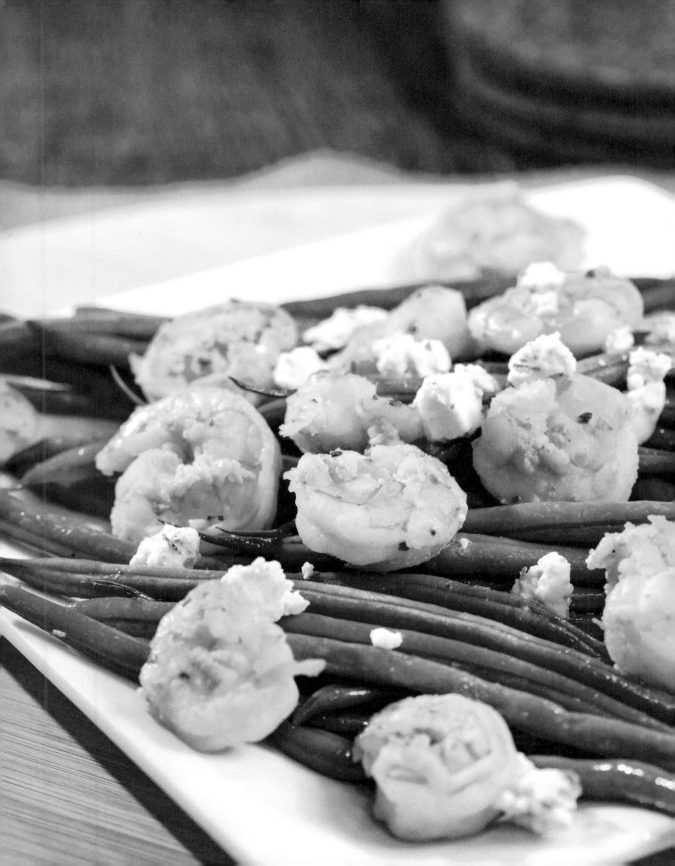

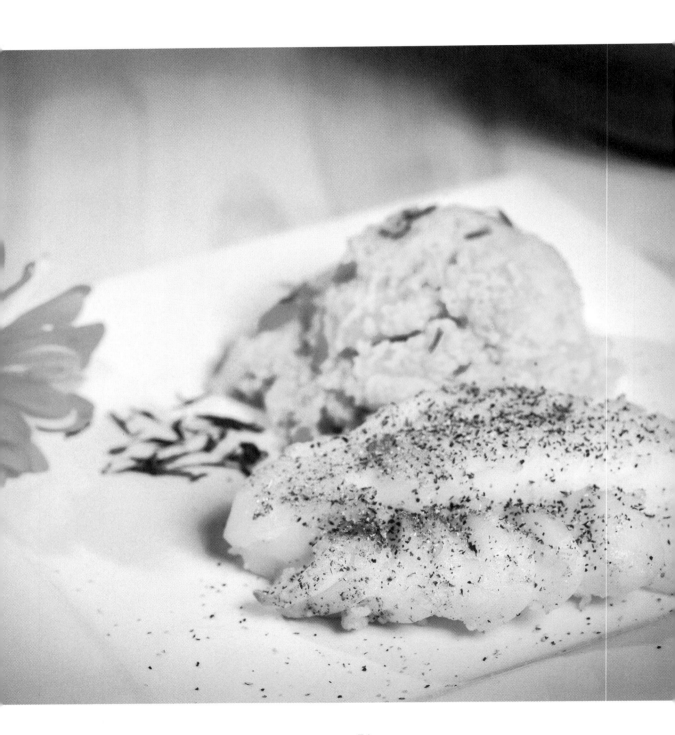

PINEAPPLE PEPPERED FLOUNDER

----

3 SERVINGS

2⅓ cups low-sodium chicken broth

1 cup whole wheat couscous

2 teaspoons extra-virgin olive oil

¼ teaspoon sea salt

¼ teaspoon freshly ground black pepper

3 (4-ounce) flounder fillets

2 cups fresh pineapple, cut into 1-inch dice

1 red bell pepper, diced

2 tablespoons chopped fresh chives

Bring 1⅓ cups of the broth to a boil in a small saucepan. Stir in the couscous.

Remove the pan from the heat immediately, cover, and let sit for 5 minutes to absorb the liquid. Set aside.

Heat the oil on medium-high heat in a large skillet.

Sprinkle the salt and black pepper on both sides of the fillets.

Place the fillets in the skillet and cook for 1 to 2 minutes per side, until golden brown. Remove from the skillet and set aside.

Add the pineapple and bell pepper to the skillet and cook over medium-high heat for 2 minutes, stirring occasionally.

Stir in the cooked couscous, chives, and the remaining 1 cup broth, and mix well.

Place the fillets on top of couscous mixture, cover with foil, and cook for 2 to 3 minutes, until the fish is tender and steaming under the foil.

Remove from the heat and serve immediately.

DAYS 29 & 30

APPLE WALNUT SPINACH SALAD

----

2 SERVINGS

1 apple, peeled, cored, and cut into bite-size pieces

4 tablespoons lemon juice

3 tablespoons extra-virgin olive oil

1 tablespoon apple cider vinegar

1 tablespoon raw honey

Salt

Freshly ground black pepper

6 cups baby spinach

1/3 cup crumbled feta cheese

1/2 cup chopped walnuts

Toss the apple with 2 tablespoons of the lemon juice.

Make the dressing: Whisk together the remaining 2 tablespoons lemon juice, oil, vinegar, and honey. Add salt and pepper to taste.

Place the spinach in a large bowl, add the dressing, and toss.

Add the apple to the salad and sprinkle the feta and walnuts on top.

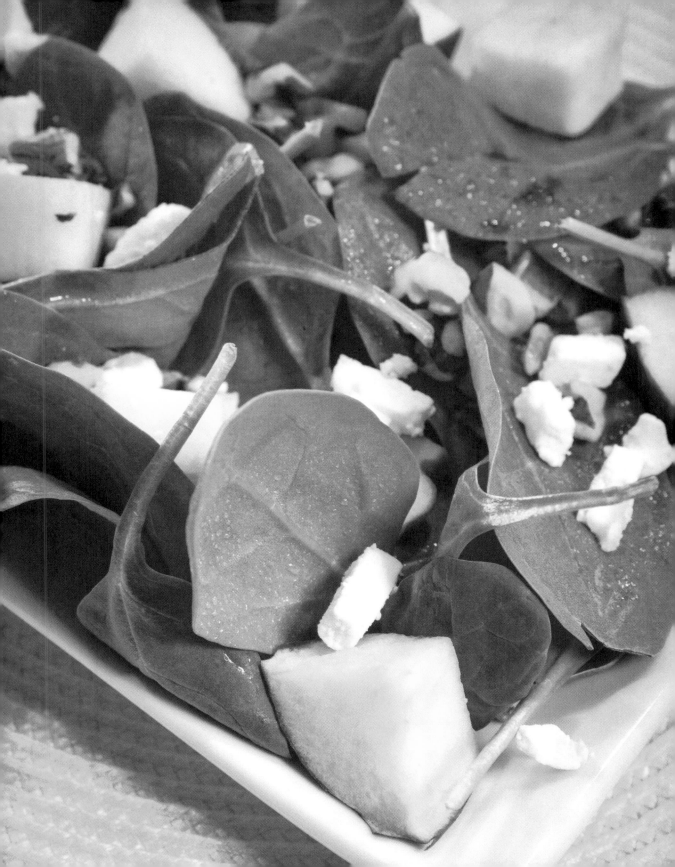

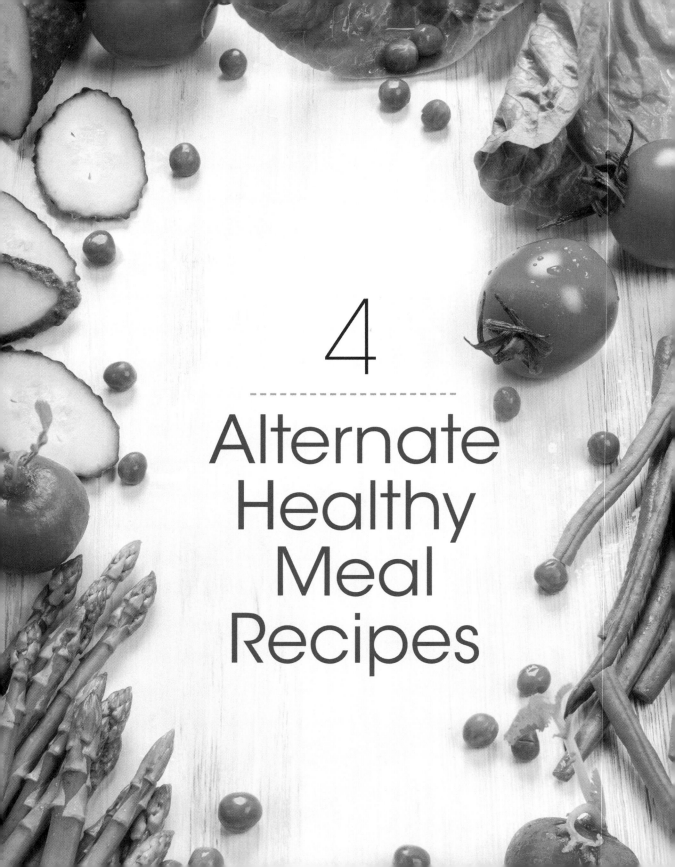

4

Alternate Healthy Meal Recipes

CRISPY BAKED CHICKEN

----

2 SERVINGS

⅓ cup dry-roasted peanuts, unsalted

1½ tablespoons garlic powder

1½ teaspoons ground ginger

8 ounces skinless chicken breast tenderloins

1 lime

Preheat the oven to 375°F.

Grind the peanuts until fine in a mini food processor.

Combine the peanuts, garlic powder, and ginger in a small bowl.

Roll the chicken in the peanut mixture until well coated.

Place the chicken on a baking sheet and squeeze lime juice over it.

Bake the chicken for 25 to 30 minutes, or until it is no longer pink in the center.

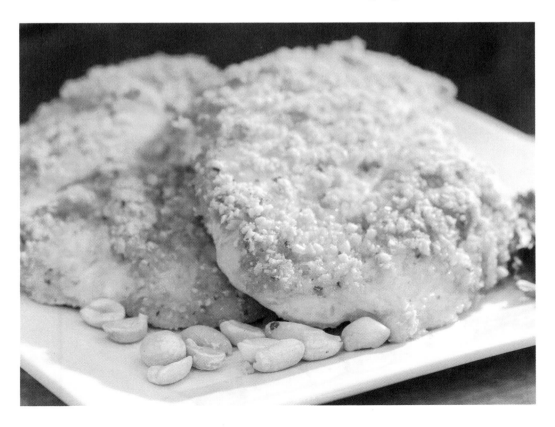

CHICKEN STEW WITH BLACK-EYED PEAS AND SWISS CHARD

---

2 SERVINGS

3 tablespoons extra-virgin olive oil

1 medium green bell pepper, stemmed, seeded, and chopped

1 small yellow or white onion, chopped

2 medium celery stalks, chopped

2 teaspoons minced fresh sage

2 teaspoons minced garlic

½ teaspoon salt

½ teaspoon freshly ground black pepper

2 to 6 dashes Tabasco sauce

12 ounces boneless, skinless chicken thighs, cut into 2-inch pieces

1 (14-ounce) can low-sodium diced tomatoes

1 cup canned black-eyed peas, rinsed and drained

½ cup low-sodium chicken broth

4 cups washed, stemmed, and chopped Swiss chard leaves (about 2 pounds with stems)

Heat the oil in a large pot over medium heat.

Add the bell pepper, onion, and celery; cook, stirring often, for 3 minutes, or until softened.

Add the sage, garlic, salt, black pepper, and Tabasco. Stir well.

Add the chicken and cook, stirring occasionally, for 2 minutes, or until it is no longer pink in the center.

Stir in the tomatoes, black-eyed peas, and broth. Raise the heat to high and bring to a boil.

Cover, reduce the heat to low, and simmer for 20 minutes.

Stir in the Swiss chard. Cover and continue cooking for 10 minutes, stirring occasionally.

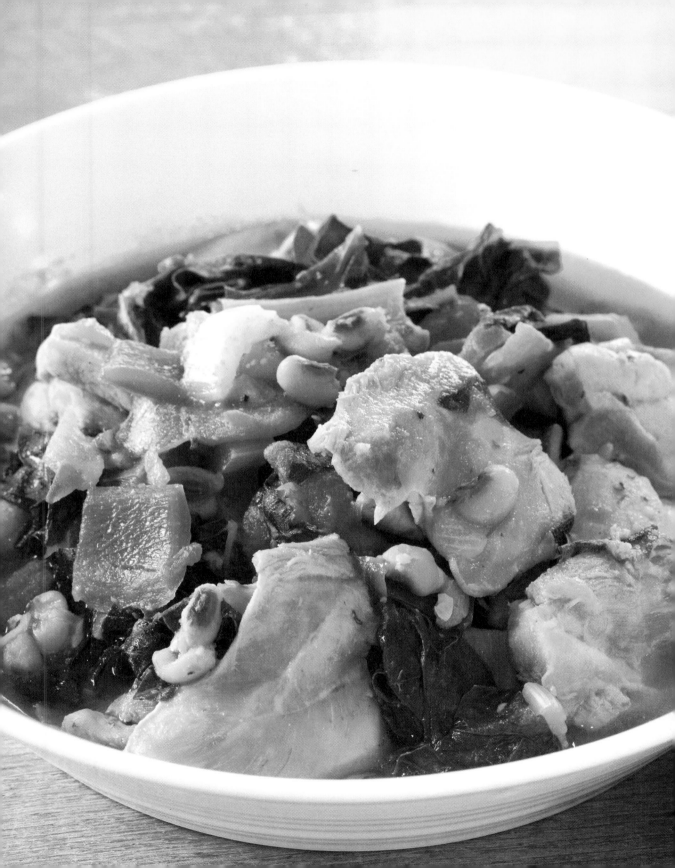

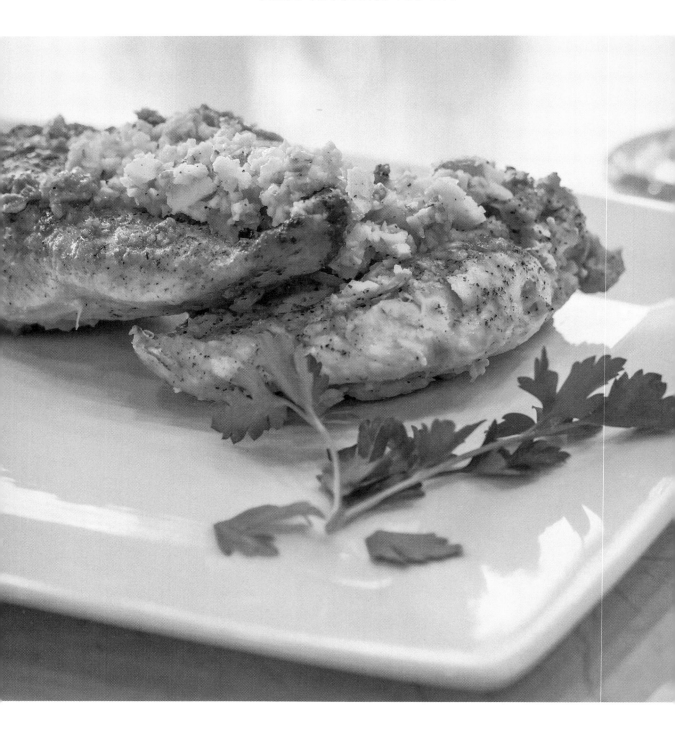

CITRUS GRILLED CHICKEN

----

2 SERVINGS

MARINADE

1 tablespoon orange zest

1 tablespoon lime zest

½ cup orange juice (no added sugar)

2 tablespoons extra-virgin olive oil

1 teaspoon minced garlic

2 (6-ounce) boneless, skinless chicken breasts

¼ teaspoon sea salt

¼ teaspoon freshly ground black pepper

2 teaspoons olive oil

Make the marinade: Combine the orange and lime zests, orange juice, the 2 tablespoons extra-virgin oil, and the garlic in a large bowl. Stir well to combine.

Add the chicken, stir to coat with the marinade, cover, and refrigerate for 30 to 45 minutes.

Remove the chicken from the marinade and sprinkle with the salt and pepper. Reserve the marinade for garnish.

Heat the 2 teaspoons olive oil in a skillet over medium-high heat and cook the chicken for 6 minutes per side, or until completely done.

VEGETABLE GUMBO

----

2 SERVINGS

2 tablespoons peanut oil

1 small yellow or white onion, chopped

1 medium green bell pepper, stemmed, seeded, and chopped

2 medium celery stalks, chopped

1 tablespoon Creole seasoning blend

1 (28-ounce) can low-sodium diced tomatoes

1 (15-ounce) can kidney beans, rinsed and drained

1 (8-ounce) package frozen sliced okra, or 2 cups sliced fresh okra

1 cup low-sodium vegetable broth

½ cup long-grain brown rice, such as basmati or Texmati

2 teaspoons gumbo filé powder

Heat the oil in a large pot or Dutch oven over medium heat.

Add the onion, bell pepper, and celery and cook, stirring often, for 4 minutes, or until softened.

Stir in the Creole seasoning and cook until fragrant, about 10 seconds.

Stir in the tomatoes, beans, okra, broth, and rice. Bring to a full simmer, stirring occasionally.

Cover, reduce the heat to low, and simmer for 45 minutes, or until the rice is tender.

Stir in the gumbo filé powder just before serving.

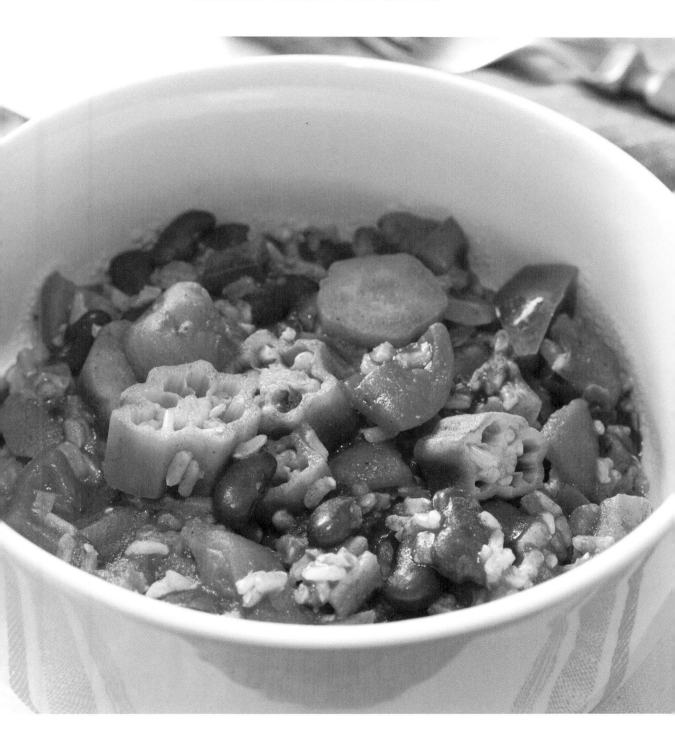

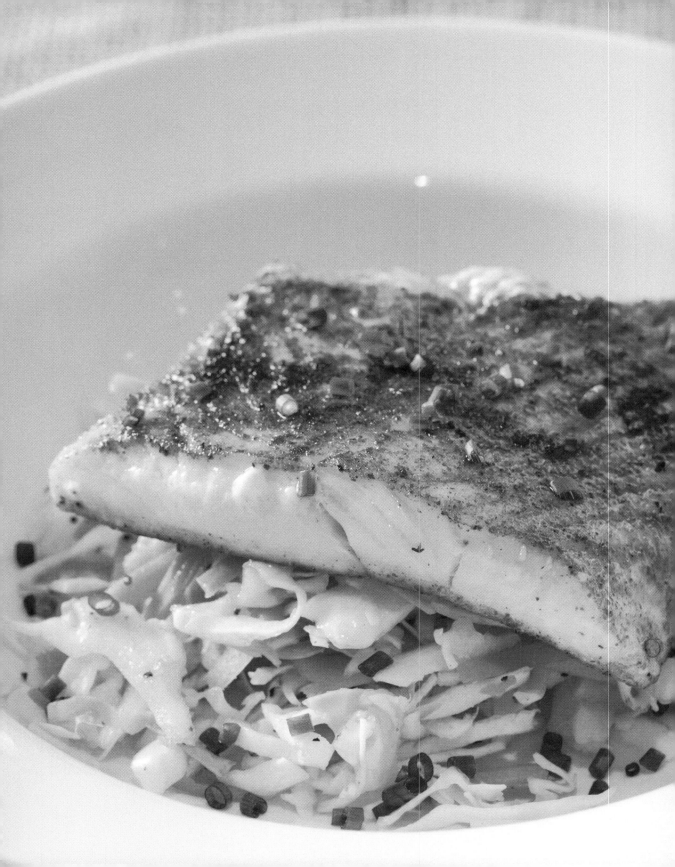

BLACKENED HALIBUT WITH SPICY COLESLAW

----

4 SERVINGS

1 (14-ounce) bag coleslaw mix

3 tablespoons lime juice

2 tablespoons raw honey

½ teaspoon ground cumin

½ teaspoon salt

2 dashes Tabasco sauce

4 (5-ounce) halibut fillets

2 teaspoons blackened seasoning blend

1 tablespoon peanut oil

Toss the coleslaw mix, lime juice, honey, cumin, salt, and Tabasco in a large bowl until well combined. Set aside.

Season the halibut fillets with the blackened seasoning.

Heat the oil in a large skillet over medium heat.

Add the fillets and cook, turning once, for 8 minutes, or until blackened and cooked through.

Divide the coleslaw among 4 serving plates. Top each with a blackened fillet.

BLUEBERRY SPINACH SALAD

----

2 SERVINGS

3 cups baby spinach, washed and dried

1 pint fresh blueberries

½ cup crumbled feta cheese

¼ cup finely chopped almonds

2 to 3 teaspoons balsamic vinaigrette

Toss together the baby spinach, blueberries, feta, and almonds in a large bowl.

Add the balsamic vinaigrette, toss, and serve.

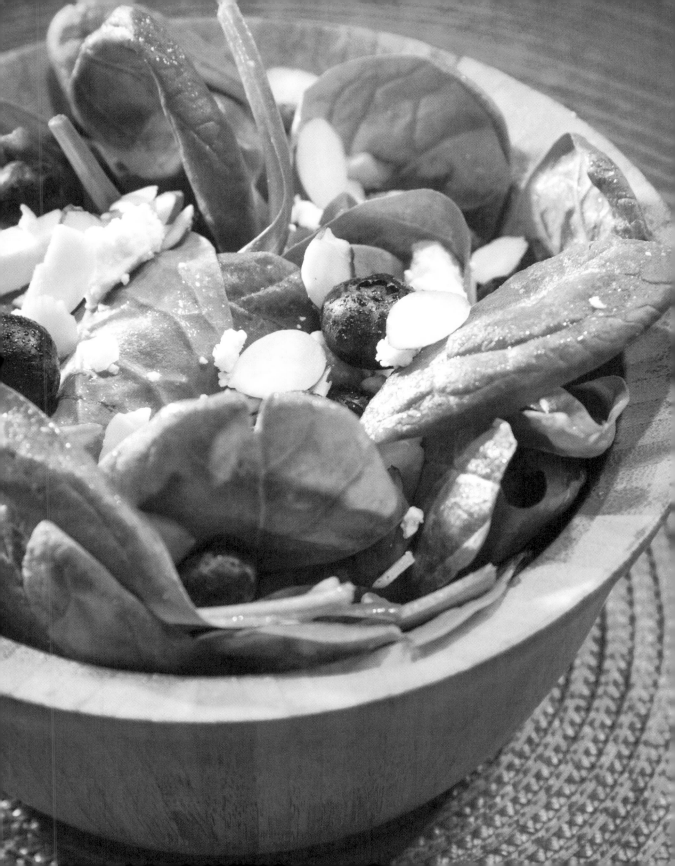

PEA SOUP

SERVES 2

10 ounces fresh or frozen peas

1 medium avocado, halved and pitted

1 cup spring water

1 cup unsweetened almond milk

2 tablespoons lime juice

½ teaspoon chili powder

Salt

Freshly ground black pepper

Blend the peas, avocado, water, almond milk, lime juice, and chili powder until very smooth in a food processor.

Place in a saucepan and heat over medium heat.

Season with salt and pepper.

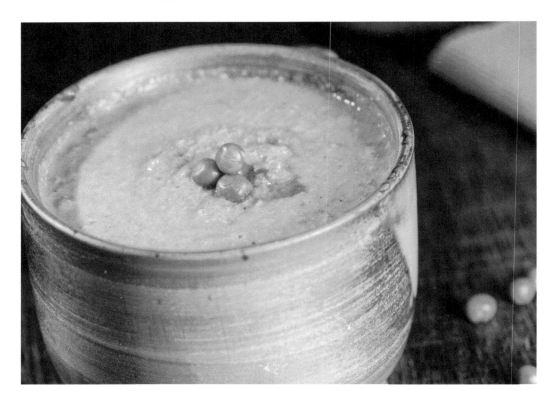

CUCUMBER TOMATO SALAD

----

2 SERVINGS

5 tomatoes (any variety)

2 small cucumbers

1 tablespoon red wine vinegar

2 tablespoons extra-virgin olive oil

¼ red onion, finely chopped

¼ teaspoon fresh basil, chopped

Salt

Freshly ground black pepper

Chop the tomatoes and cucumbers into bite-size pieces and combine in a bowl.

Combine the vinegar, oil, onion, and basil in another bowl.

Add the salt and pepper to taste.

Pour the salad dressing over the tomatoes and serve.

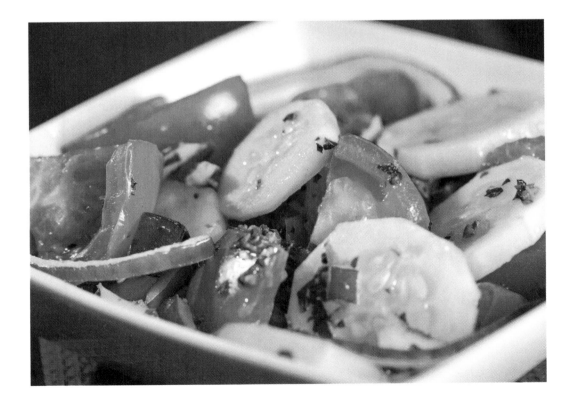

JERK SHRIMP STEW

----

2 SERVINGS

1 tablespoon coconut oil

5 medium scallions, thinly sliced

1 teaspoon minced garlic

1 pound medium shrimp (about 30 per pound), peeled and deveined

1 red bell pepper, stemmed, seeded, and cut into ½-inch strips

1 cup fresh green beans, stemmed and cut into 1-inch pieces

1 tablespoon jerk seasoning blend

1 teaspoon apple cider vinegar

½ cup light coconut milk

¼ cup low-sodium vegetable broth

Melt the coconut oil in a large saucepan over medium heat.

Add the scallions and garlic, and cook, stirring often, for 1 minute.

Add the shrimp and cook, stirring occasionally, for 3 minutes, or until pink.

Add the bell pepper, green beans, and jerk seasoning. Cook for 1 minute, or until fragrant.

Stir in the vinegar, then pour in the coconut milk and broth.

Bring to a simmer, stirring occasionally. Cover, reduce the heat, and simmer for 5 minutes to blend the flavors.

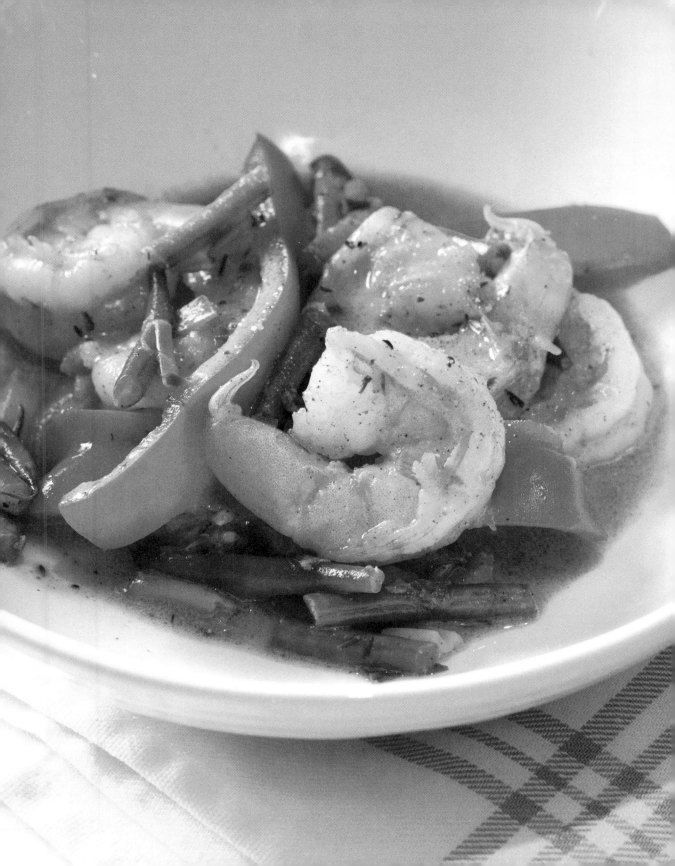

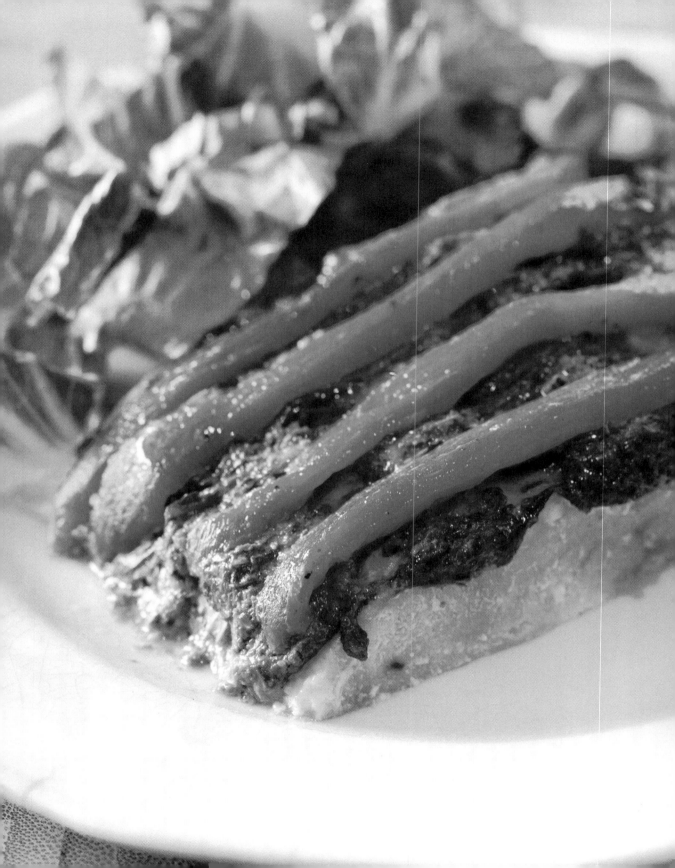

PESTO ROASTED SALMON

4 SERVINGS

1 cup packed fresh basil leaves

3 tablespoons chopped pecans

3 tablespoons juice from a jar of roasted red pepper

1 medium garlic clove, peeled

1 teaspoon dried oregano

½ teaspoon salt

½ teaspoon freshly ground black pepper

1 tablespoon extra-virgin olive oil

4 (5-ounce) skin-on salmon fillets

1 roasted red pepper (from a jar), cut into thin strips

Preheat the oven to 450°F.

Puree the basil, pecans, red pepper juice, garlic, oregano, salt, and pepper in a blender or a small food processor until it forms a paste.

Grease a 9 x 13-inch baking pan with the oil. Place the salmon skin side down in the pan.

Spread the basil mixture evenly over the fillets. Lay the pepper strips on top of each fillet.

Roast for 15 minutes, or until cooked through.

TAMARI-GLAZED SALMON

----

2 SERVINGS

¼ cup tamari soy sauce (low-sodium)

2 tablespoons raw honey

1 tablespoon rice vinegar

1 tablespoon ground ginger

¼ teaspoon cayenne pepper

⅛ teaspoon freshly ground black pepper

2 large salmon fillets

Preheat the oven to 425°F.

Line a roasting pan or baking sheet with aluminum foil.

Combine the tamari, honey, vinegar, ginger, cayenne, and black pepper in a large bowl.

Add the salmon, turning the pieces over in the marinade. Cover the bowl and refrigerate for 2 to 3 hours.

Place the salmon in the roasting pan, skin side down and bake in the oven for 15 to 20 minutes, until it flakes easily.

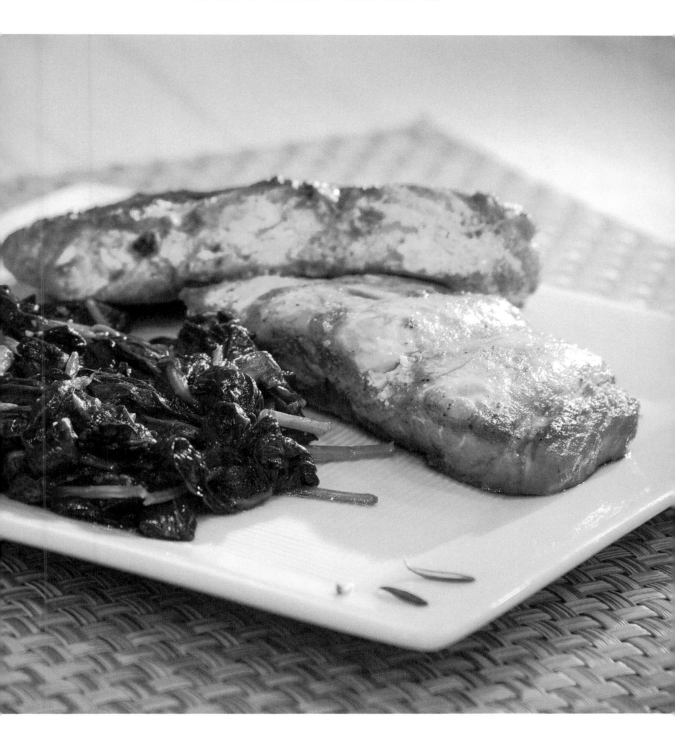

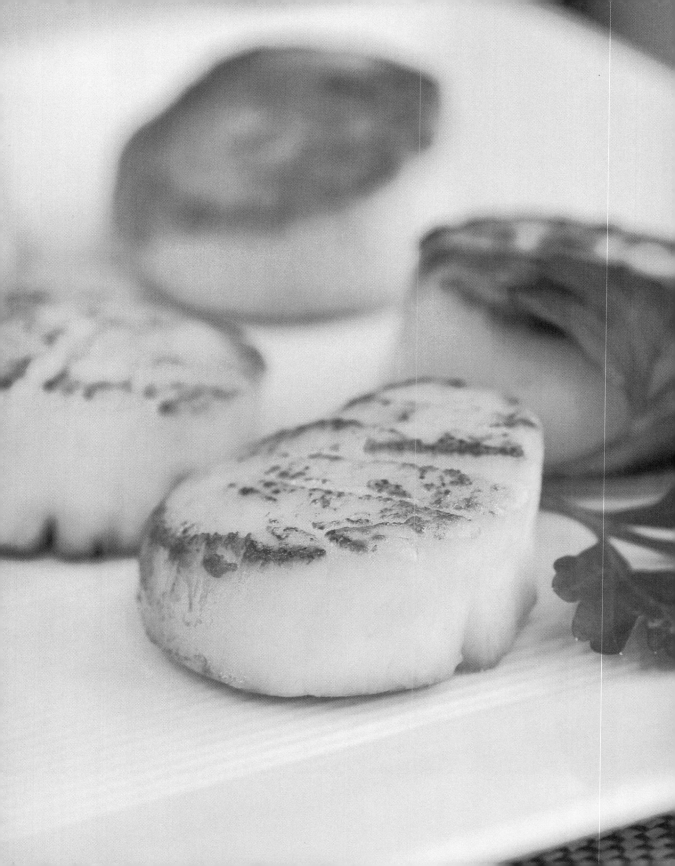

SCALLOPS WITH LEMON SAUCE

----

4 SERVINGS

4 tablespoons fresh lemon juice

½ cup fresh parsley

2 garlic cloves

1 teaspoon sea salt, plus more

½ teaspoon freshly ground black pepper, plus more

½ cup extra-virgin olive oil

Cooking spray

3 pounds sea scallops, preferably dry sea scallops which are more pure

Make the sauce: Combine the lemon juice, parsley, garlic, salt, and pepper in a small bowl. Whisk in the oil and set aside.

Coat a skillet with cooking spray and heat over medium heat.

Rinse and pat the scallops dry and sprinkle with salt and pepper.

Put the scallops in the skillet and cook for 2 to 3 minutes on each side.

Remove the scallops from the pan and spoon the lemon sauce over them.

COLLARD GREENS STEW WITH BLACK-EYED PEAS

----

2 SERVINGS

4 cups low-sodium vegetable broth

1 pound collard greens, cleaned and chopped

1 (15-ounce) can diced tomatoes (no added salt)

1 (15-ounce) can cooked black-eyed peas, rinsed and drained

Freshly ground black pepper

Salt

Combine the broth and 2 cups of water in a large saucepan and bring to a boil.

Add the collard greens, cover, reduce the heat to low, and simmer for 15 minutes.

Add the tomatoes and return to a simmer.

Cover and cook until the tomatoes are tender, 3 to 5 minutes.

Stir in the black-eyed peas and simmer for 2 to 4 minutes, until thoroughly heated.

Season with salt and pepper, and serve immediately.

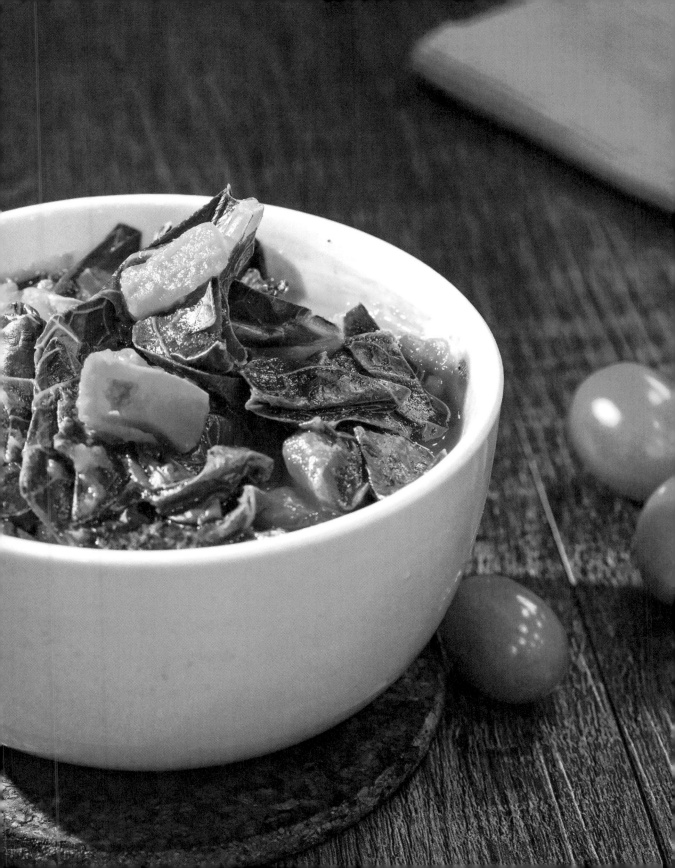

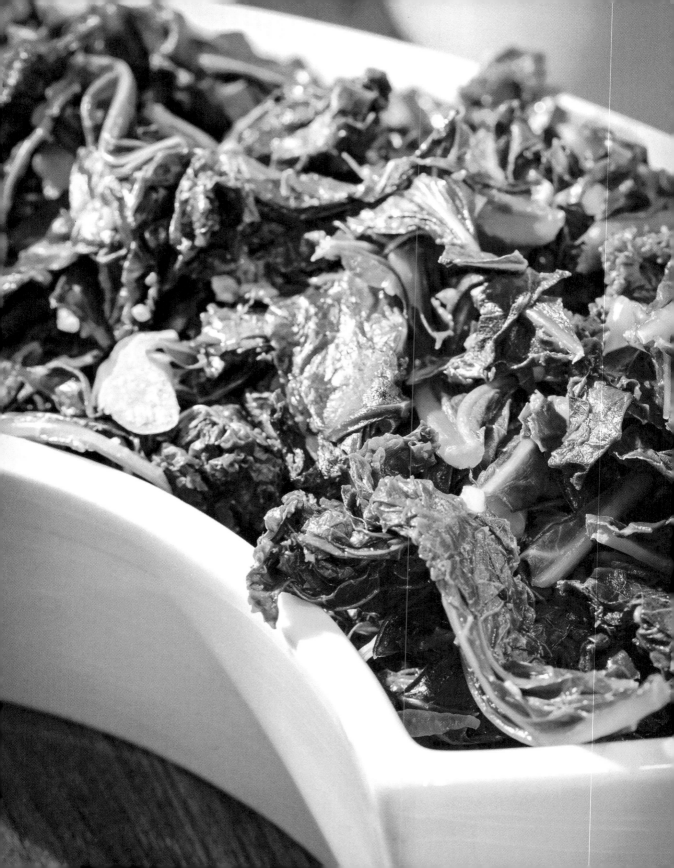

GREEN LEAFY STIR-FRY

----

2 SERVINGS

1 pound dark green leafy veggies (such as collards, kale, spinach, mustard greens, dandelion greens, chard, etc.)

2 tablespoons extra-virgin olive oil

3 cloves garlic, minced

½ small red onion, minced

⅛ teaspoon powdered ginger, or ½-inch piece of fresh ginger, peeled and grated

1 tablespoon dry sherry

2 teaspoons low-sodium soy sauce

Pinch of stevia

Chop the greens into small pieces, wash, and dry them.

Heat the oil over medium-high heat in a large nonstick skillet. Add the greens, garlic, onion, ginger, sherry, and soy sauce. Sprinkle with water to keep the greens from burning.

Cook, stirring constantly for a few minutes, or until the stems begin to soften.

Add the stevia to taste and serve.

ALMOND-CRUSTED BAKED CHICKEN

----

2 SERVINGS

1 cup almonds

2 teaspoons oregano

¼ cup Parmesan cheese

1 teaspoon sea salt

Freshly ground black pepper

1 teaspoon thyme

15 ounces chicken breast tenderloins

2 egg whites, lightly beaten

Preheat the oven to 350°F. Line a baking sheet with parchment paper.

Make the almond crust: Process the almonds, oregano, Parmesan, salt, pepper, and thyme in a food processor until the mixture is finely ground

Place the chicken on a plate. Put the egg whites in one bowl and the almond mixture in another.

Gently roll each piece of chicken first in the egg whites, then in the almond mixture, and place it on the baking sheet.

Bake for 25 to 30 minutes.

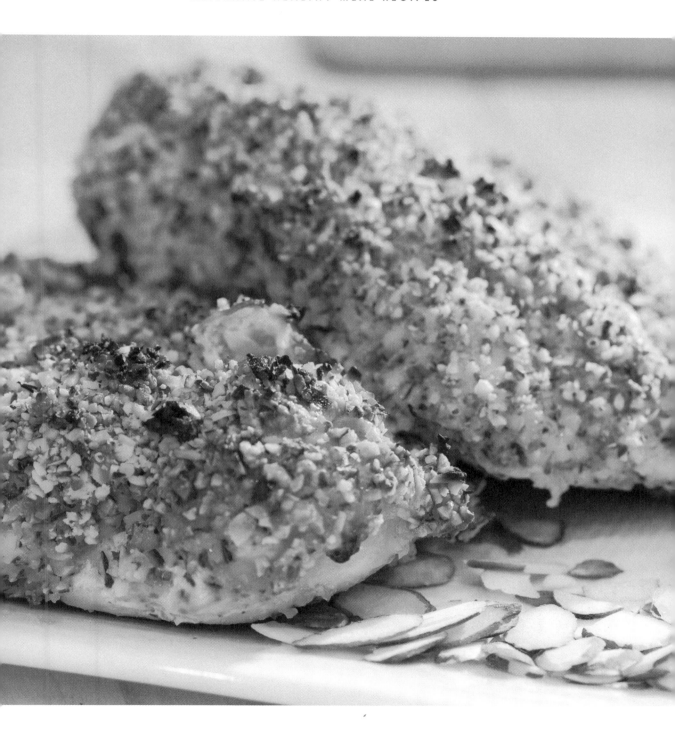

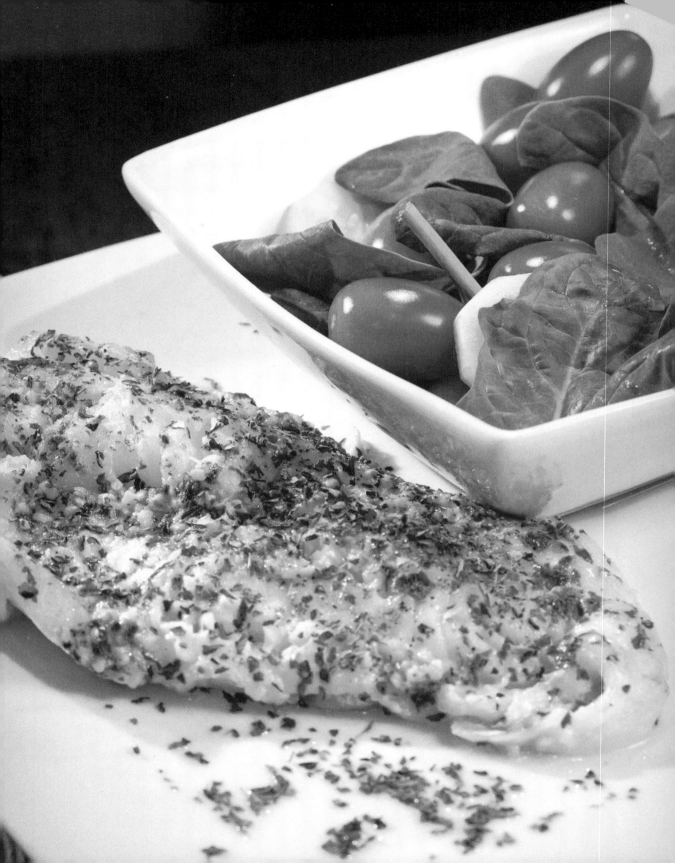

BAKED HALIBUT

----

2 SERVINGS

2 (6-ounce) boneless halibut fillets

1 teaspoon extra-virgin olive oil

2 small garlic cloves, minced

2 teaspoons lemon zest

2 tablespoons fresh lemon juice

1 tablespoon chopped parsley

Dash of sea salt

Freshly ground black pepper

Preheat the oven to 400°F.

Place the halibut skin side down and drizzle with the oil in a large nonstick baking dish.

Combine the garlic, lemon zest, lemon juice, and parsley in a bowl and mix well.

Coat the halibut with the garlic mixture and season with salt and pepper.

Bake for 13 to 15 minutes, until the halibut flakes easily.

5

Sweet Treats (Desserts)

A sweet indulgence every now and again is acceptable, particularly when you're drinking smoothies and eating clean otherwise.

OATMEAL-RAISIN COOKIES

MAKES 15 COOKIES

2 ripe bananas, mashed

1 cup quick-cooking oats, uncooked

¼ cup raisins

¼ cup shredded coconut, chopped nuts, or unsweetened chocolate chips

Preheat the oven to 350°F.

Combine the bananas, oats, raisins, and coconut. Stir with a wooden spoon in a bowl.

Drop the batter by the tablespoonful onto a cookie sheet and flatten.

Bake for 15 to 20 minutes, or until the edges are brown.

Remove the cookies from the cookie sheet and let cool on a cooling rack.

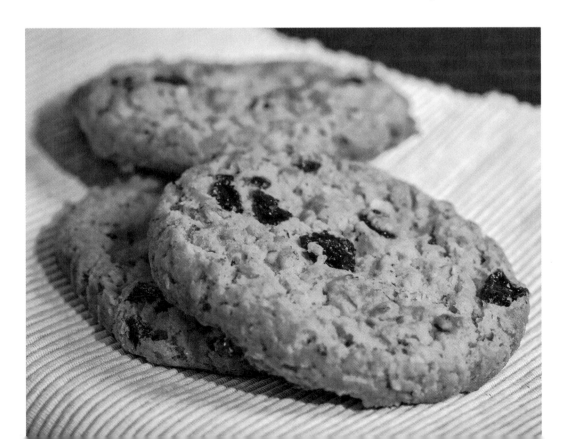

MANGO BANANA NUT
ICE CREAM

----

4 bananas, sliced and frozen

1 ripe mango, or 2 large peaches

¼ cup sliced almonds,
for topping

Place the bananas and mango in a blender and blend until smooth. If it's too loose, add more bananas.

Place in serving bowls, sprinkle the almonds on top, and serve immediately.

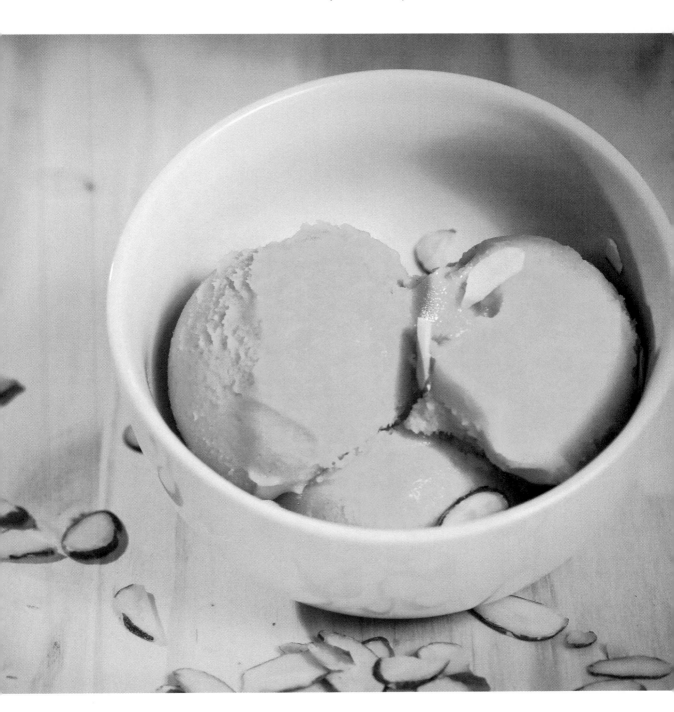

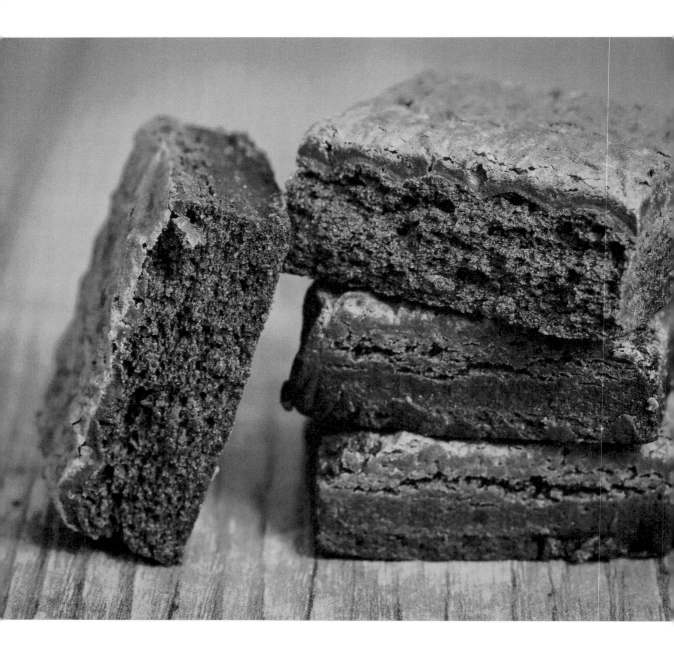

COCONUT BROWNIES

⅓ cup coconut flour

⅓ cup unsweetened cocoa powder

⅓ cup coconut oil

5 whole eggs

½ cup maple syrup

2 teaspoons pure vanilla extract

1 cup chopped walnuts (optional)

Preheat the oven to 350°F. Grease an 8-inch square baking pan.

Whisk together the coconut flour and cocoa powder in a mixing bowl.

Whisk in the oil, eggs, maple syrup, and vanilla, and blend well.

Add the walnuts, if using.

Pour the batter into the baking pan and bake for about 30 minutes.

Allow to cool well in the pan before serving or the brownies will fall apart.

STRAWBERRY ALMOND DELIGHT

1 pound strawberries, sliced

¼ cup chopped almonds

Juice of ½ lemon

¼ teaspoon pure vanilla extract

1 tablespoon honey

Dash of cinnamon

Combine the strawberries, almonds, lemon juice, vanilla, honey, and cinnamon in a large bowl. Stir well and serve.

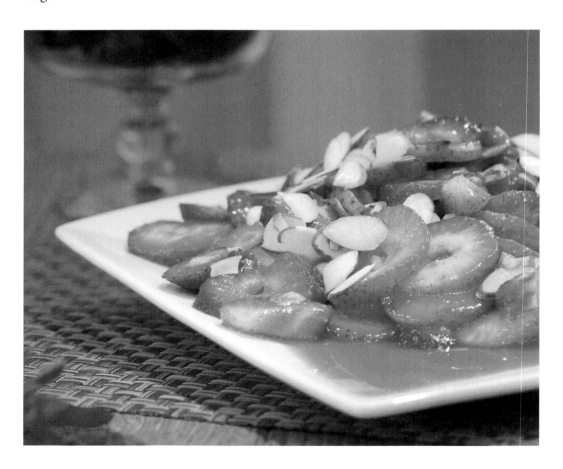

BANANA STRAWBERRY ICE CREAM

----

4 large bananas, sliced and frozen

2 cups frozen strawberries

½ cup almond milk (unsweetened vanilla almond milk is ideal)

Place the bananas, strawberries, and almond milk in a blender and blend, stirring frequently, until it has a creamy consistency.

Be careful not to overblend as that will cause the ice cream to melt.

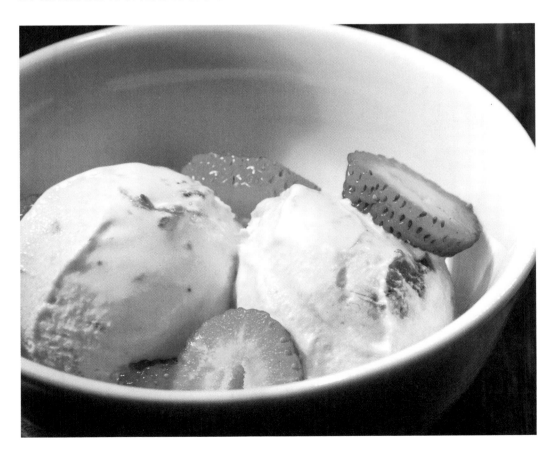

CHOCOLATE CHIP COOKIES

MAKES 15 COOKIES

⅓ cup cooked oatmeal

⅛ cup whole wheat pastry flour

3 tablespoons raw honey

1 teaspoon pure vanilla extract

1 teaspoon cinnamon

½ cup unsweetened chocolate chips

⅔ cup pecans

Preheat the oven to 325°F. Line a cookie sheet with parchment paper.

Place the oatmeal, flour, honey, vanilla, and cinnamon in a food processor, and blend to combine.

Using a spatula, scrape the dough into a mixing bowl. Stir in the chocolate chips and pecans.

Drop the dough by the tablespoonful onto the cookie sheet and bake for 20 minutes.

Remove the cookies from the cookie sheet and let cool on a baking rack.

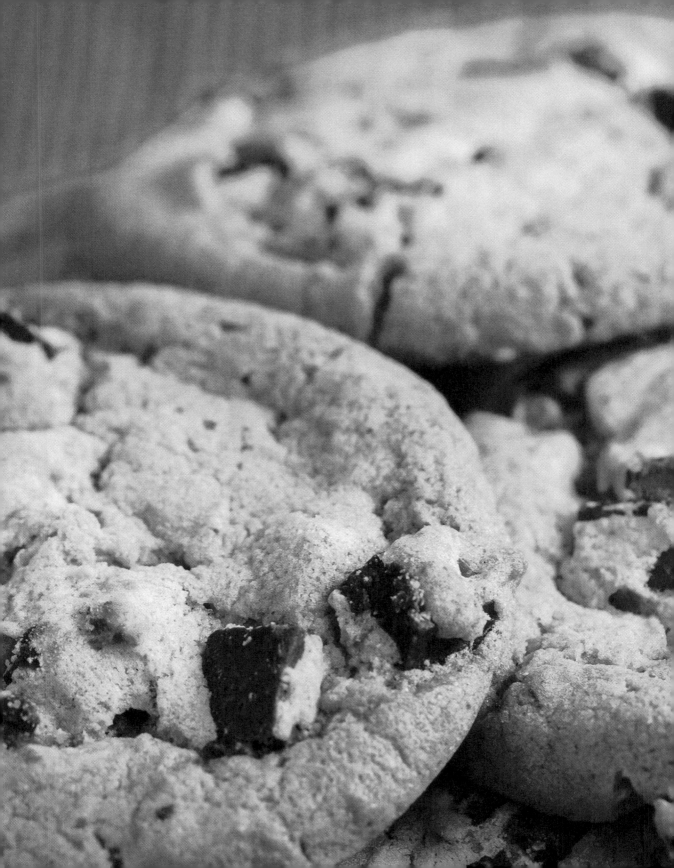

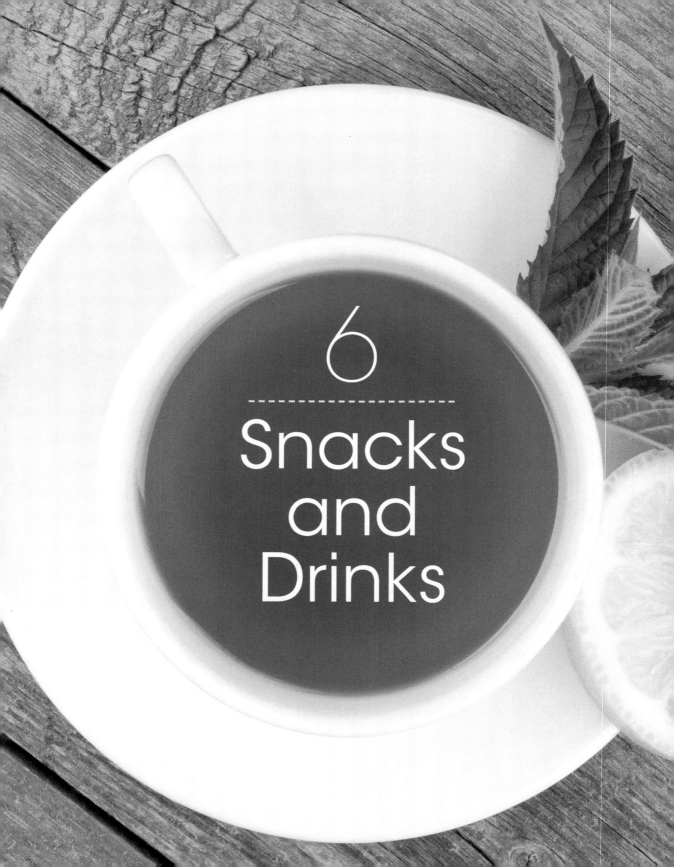

6

Snacks
and
Drinks

Snacks are critical for success. It's important to eat snacks every few hours to ensure that you keep your metabolism revved up and to avoid feeling hungry. Because we don't want you to be diet-minded, we suggest you learn to snack in moderation.

SNACKS

Here are some great snack options:

- apples
- raw veggies (celery, carrots, cucumbers, and broccoli)
- raw or unsalted nuts and seeds (only a handful)
- hard-boiled eggs
- popcorn, lightly salted
- kale chips
- protein bars (nondairy)
- hummus
- unsweetened peanut butter (less than 3 grams of sugar)

DRINKS

There are many healthy drink options that you can enjoy during the 30-Day Meal Plan:

- water (spring or alkaline)
- ACV Detox Water (described in Chapter 10)
- detox, herbal, or green tea
- herbal coffee, such as Teeccino coffee, or 1 cup of regular coffee

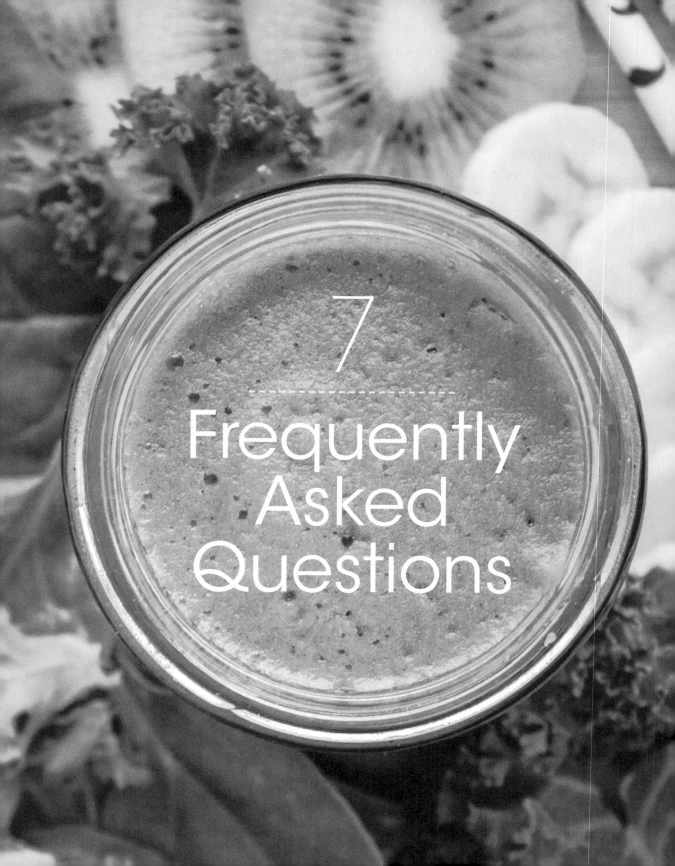

7

Frequently
Asked
Questions

H̶ere are some of the most frequently asked questions (FAQs) about the 30-Day Meal Plan.

How is this program different from the 10-Day Green Smoothie Cleanse?

➤ The 10-Day Green Smoothie Cleanse is a more intense detox regimen, with a lot more restrictions and intense detox symptoms. With the 30-Day Program, you still get to detox your body, but you also get to eat hot meals every day, enjoy coffee and green tea, and even have a special treat (dessert) each week. You will also have fewer and less intense detox symptoms because you're detoxing more slowly over a 30-day period. However, on both programs, you'll experience weight loss, improved energy, better digestion, less bloating, and improved mental clarity.

What if I want to make my own healthy meals?

➤ If you want to make your own meals beyond those provided in this book, please be sure that they are clean, healthy, high-protein meals. Additionally, be sure you're also avoiding the "do not eat" items in all of your healthy meal recipes. If you follow those rules, you can definitely swap out the recommended healthy meals for some of your own favorite healthy meals.

If I just finished the 10-Day Green Smoothie Cleanse, can I still do the 30-Day Meal Plan?

➤ Absolutely! The 30-Day Program is designed to follow the 10-Day Green Smoothie Cleanse. However, remember to always "break the cleanse" once you finish the 10-Day Green Smoothie Cleanse. To break the cleanse, allow three days to reintroduce whole foods into your diet. Salads are a good way to start. Make delightful salad dressings to please your palate. Continue drinking your smoothies and listen to your body to see what foods work well for you.

What do I do after the 30 days?

➤ Once you complete the 30 days, feel free to join us in the VIP Group (for more information on the VIP group see Appendix B), which offers long-term accountability and motivation for permanent weight loss. The VIP Group is where you can learn more about my DHEMM System and other principles for weight loss, such as balancing your hormones for weight loss and how to have the right mind-set to keep the weight off.

How many snacks can I have per day?

➤ Don't think diet, think detox cleanse, so calories and serving sizes are not the focus. There are no hard-and-fast rules. But you should snack in moderation when you're hungry. Trying to eat by counting calories and serving sizes won't create a lifestyle change. You'll just be on a diet for life. I don't know about you, but I'm done with dieting! Ninety-five percent of people who lose weight on a fad diet gain it back in three to five years. So, you're changing your eating habits for life, retraining your taste buds to desire and crave healthier foods! Having said all that, the one caution I would give is on nuts and seeds. They are healthy fats but fats nonetheless. They can work against you if you eat too many. When snacking on nuts and seeds, take only a handful!

Should I take my medications or supplements during the 30-Day Meal Plan?

➤ You should talk to your doctor before starting this program. I am not a medical doctor. You should never stop taking any medications prescribed by a doctor. Whether or not you continue to take your current vitamin supplements during the cleanse is up to you.

What if I'm allergic to one of the fruits in the recipe?

➤ If you're allergic to any fruit in a recipe, just leave it out and add more of the other fruits to make up for it.

How long will my smoothie keep?

➤ It is always ideal to drink your smoothie the same day you blend it to ensure that you get maximum nutrition from it. However, if you are busy or for some other reason can't make them fresh, they will keep extremely well for up to two days in the refrigerator. A glass jar with a lid is ideal to safely store your smoothies. Covering your green smoothies with a tight lid minimizes oxidation and absorption of other smells from the refrigerator. Additionally, making the smoothies the night before is okay if it helps you stay on track.

Can I use agave or honey instead of stevia in the smoothies?

➤ Agave is okay in moderation, but if you're interested in weight loss, stevia is the number-one sweetener. The way to think about sweeteners is how much they cause insulin spikes, because that determines how much they will cause fat storage in the body. Foods are given glycemic index (GI) ratings according to how much they cause insulin spikes. Stevia is a 0 (which is ideal). Agave is a 20. Honey is about a 30. Brown sugar/raw sugar is a 65. And white refined sugar is an 80. So that gives you some perspective. I have four friends who all use different brands of stevia, and none of us like the others' stevia because they all taste different. If you think you don't like stevia, try another brand. You might find you just don't like the brand you've been using.

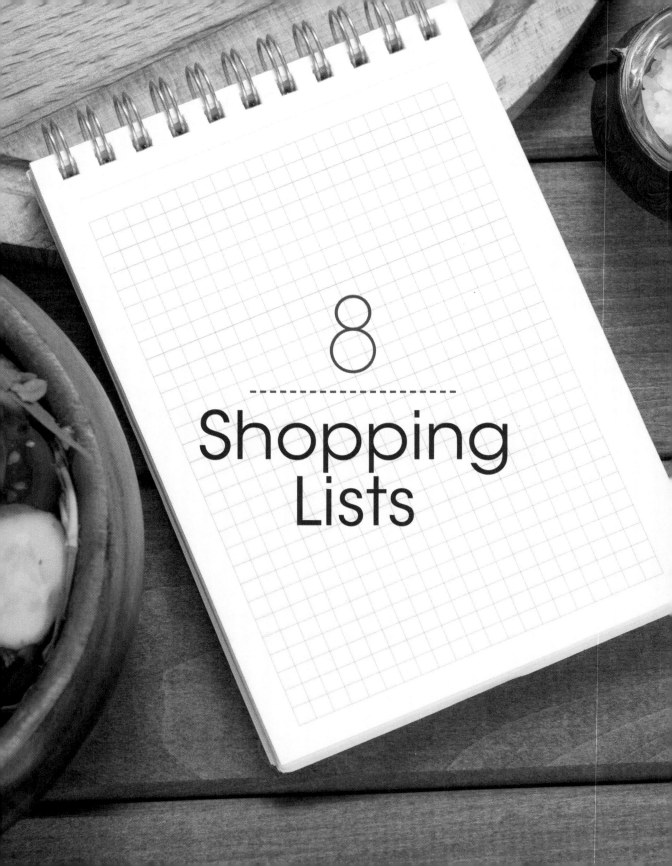

8
Shopping Lists

Green Smoothie Recipes

DAYS 1–10

- ☐ 4 bananas
- ☐ 3 apples
- ☐ 4 ounces fresh or frozen seedless grapes
- ☐ 40 ounces frozen peach slices
- ☐ 64 ounces frozen blueberries
- ☐ 24 ounces frozen strawberries
- ☐ 32 ounces frozen mixed berries
- ☐ 82 ounces frozen pineapple chunks
- ☐ 54 ounces fresh spinach leaves
- ☐ 6 ounces fresh baby kale
- ☐ Stevia sweetener (packets)

- ☐ Bag of ground flaxseeds (often in the vitamin section)
- ☐ Snacks (such as apples, carrots, celery, broccoli, cucumber, etc.)
- ☐ Raw or unsalted nuts and seeds to snack on
- ☐ Drinks: detox tea (any flavor), herbal tea, green tea, caffeine-free herbal coffee, spring water (lemon water if desired)
- ☐ Optional: Nondairy/plant-based protein powder, such as Nutiva Hemp Protein, RAW Protein by Garden of Life, or Sun Warrior protein

Green Smoothie Recipes

DAYS 11–20

- ☐ 7 bananas
- ☐ 6 apples
- ☐ 1 orange
- ☐ 4 ounces fresh or frozen seedless grapes
- ☐ 48 ounces frozen peach slices
- ☐ 24 ounces frozen blueberries
- ☐ 28 ounces frozen strawberries
- ☐ 16 ounces frozen mixed berries
- ☐ 48 ounces frozen pineapple chunks
- ☐ 28 ounces frozen mango chunks
- ☐ 54 ounces fresh spinach leaves
- ☐ 10 ounces spring mix lettuce leaves
- ☐ Stevia sweetener (packets)
- ☐ Bag of ground flaxseeds (often in vitamin section)
- ☐ Snacks (such as apples, carrots, celery, broccoli, cucumber, etc.)
- ☐ Raw or unsalted nuts and seeds to snack on
- ☐ Drinks: detox tea (any flavor), herbal tea, green tea, caffeine-free herbal coffee, spring water (lemon water if desired)
- ☐ Optional: Nondairy/plant-based protein powder, such as Nutiva Hemp Protein, RAW Protein by Garden of Life, or Sun Warrior protein

Green Smoothie Recipes

DAYS 21-30

- ☐ 3 bananas
- ☐ 3 apples
- ☐ 4 ounces fresh or frozen seedless grapes
- ☐ 56 ounces frozen peach slices
- ☐ 44 ounces frozen blueberries
- ☐ 24 ounces frozen strawberries
- ☐ 28 ounces frozen mixed berries
- ☐ 80 ounces frozen pineapple chunks
- ☐ 12 ounces frozen mango chunks
- ☐ 54 ounces fresh spinach leaves
- ☐ 10 ounces fresh baby kale leaves

- ☐ Stevia sweetener (packets)
- ☐ Bag of ground flaxseeds (often in vitamin section)
- ☐ Snacks (such as apples, carrots, celery, broccoli, cucumber, etc.)
- ☐ Raw or unsalted nuts and seeds to snack on
- ☐ Drinks: detox tea (any flavor), herbal tea, green tea, caffeine-free herbal coffee, spring water (lemon water if desired)
- ☐ Optional: Nondairy/plant-based protein powder, such as Nutiva Hemp Protein, RAW Protein by Garden of Life, or Sun Warrior protein

Healthy Dinner Recipes

DAYS 1-10

- ☐ 12 ounces salmon fillets
- ☐ 2 pounds skin-on, bone-in chicken quarters
- ☐ 1 pound boneless, skinless chicken breasts
- ☐ 1 pound sea scallops
- ☐ 1 small cauliflower head
- ☐ 2 medium bell peppers, red and yellow
- ☐ 2 heads romaine lettuce hearts
- ☐ baby spinach (5 cups)
- ☐ broccoli (1 cup)
- ☐ baby carrots (1 cup)
- ☐ baby kale (6 cups)
- ☐ strawberries, hulled and sliced (1 cup)
- ☐ 1 lemon
- ☐ 1 red onion

- ☐ 1 jar roasted red peppers
- ☐ black beans (1½ cups)
- ☐ Parmesan cheese
- ☐ pumpkin seeds (¼ cup)
- ☐ extra-virgin olive oil (small bottle)
- ☐ coconut oil (small bottle)
- ☐ fresh dill
- ☐ sea salt
- ☐ ground black pepper
- ☐ garlic salt
- ☐ lemon pepper
- ☐ Cajun seasoning
- ☐ red wine vinegar (small bottle)
- ☐ balsamic vinegar (small bottle)
- ☐ Dijon mustard (small jar)
- ☐ agave (small bottle)
- ☐ Caesar dressing (low-sodium)

Healthy Dinner Recipes

DAYS 11–20

- ☐ ⅔ pound boneless grilled chicken breast
- ☐ 1 pound fresh precooked shrimp
- ☐ 1 pound jumbo shrimp
- ☐ 1 pound turkey cutlets
- ☐ 3 pounds collard greens
- ☐ baby spinach (8 cups)
- ☐ black-eyed peas (2 cans)
- ☐ tomato paste, no sugar added (1 small can)
- ☐ Parmesan cheese
- ☐ chopped walnuts (¾ cup)
- ☐ pecans (¼ cup)
- ☐ extra-virgin olive oil (small bottle)
- ☐ dry white wine, domestic (small bottle)
- ☐ red wine vinegar (small bottle)
- ☐ apple cider vinegar (small bottle)

- ☐ 1 garlic head
- ☐ 2 red onions
- ☐ 3 small zucchini, or 2 large
- ☐ 1 apple
- ☐ 1 lemon
- ☐ lemon juice (small bottle)
- ☐ Dijon mustard (small jar)
- ☐ sea salt
- ☐ ground black pepper
- ☐ crushed red pepper flakes
- ☐ garlic powder
- ☐ dried basil
- ☐ fresh parsley
- ☐ nutmeg
- ☐ coconut oil spray
- ☐ parchment paper

Healthy Dinner Recipes

DAYS 21-30

- ☐ 1 pound large shrimp
- ☐ 1 pound trout fillets
- ☐ 12 ounces flounder fillets
- ☐ baby spinach (12 cups)
- ☐ 1 pound fresh green beans
- ☐ 4 plum tomatoes
- ☐ 3 small red onions
- ☐ 2 garlic heads
- ☐ 2 large shallots
- ☐ 1 red bell pepper
- ☐ fresh pineapple (2 cups)
- ☐ chickpeas (1 cup)
- ☐ chopped walnuts (½ cup)
- ☐ 1 apple
- ☐ 1 lemon
- ☐ lemon juice (small bottle)
- ☐ key lime juice (small bottle)
- ☐ raw honey (small bottle)

- ☐ low-sodium chicken broth (3 cans)
- ☐ apple cider vinegar (small bottle)
- ☐ grapeseed oil (small bottle)
- ☐ extra-virgin olive oil (small bottle)
- ☐ crumbled garlic or herb feta cheese (about 1 cup)
- ☐ whole wheat couscous (1 cup)
- ☐ dried rosemary
- ☐ fresh chives
- ☐ fresh ginger
- ☐ fresh thyme
- ☐ garlic salt
- ☐ sea salt
- ☐ ground black pepper
- ☐ ground cumin
- ☐ aluminum foil

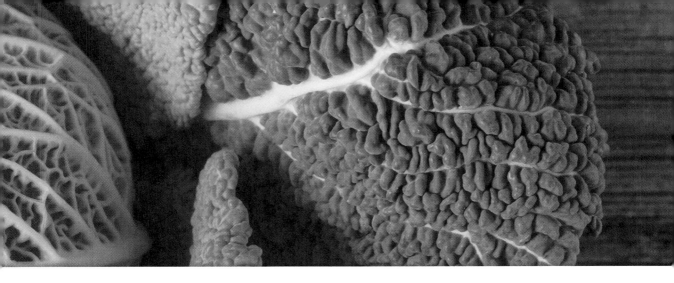

PART 2

DETOXIFICATION FOR WEIGHT LOSS AND GREAT HEALTH

After your body utilizes nutrients from the food you eat, it must dispose of the un-used food particles and waste produced by the digestive process. Without proper and complete elimination, undigested food can back up and leave toxins and waste in your body. Detoxification is the process of cleansing and reducing the toxic overload that currently resides in your body. Because there are so many toxins in your cells, tissues, and organs, you detoxify to bring them out of hiding so they can be eliminated from the body.

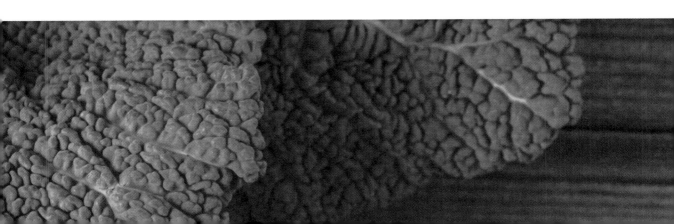

As detailed in Part 4, where I address the Detox, Hormonal Balance, Eat, Mental Mastery and Move (DHEMM) system, there are many factors that contribute to weight gain, and the one that is most overlooked by traditional diets is toxic overload. People often have difficulty losing weight because their bodies are full of toxins. The more toxins you take in or get exposed to every day, the more toxins you store as fat cells in the body. Toxins stored in fat cells are difficult to get rid of through dieting and working out. You must first detoxify the body to get rid of those fat cells. This is why detoxification has to be a primary component of any weight-loss plan if you want to lose weight permanently.

Traditional diets so often don't work because they don't address the toxic waste in the body. Counting calories does not detoxify and cleanse the body. Weight loss won't be permanent if your body's systems are sluggish or impacted with acidic waste or toxins. Once you rid your body of toxins, you will be able to better metabolize the food you eat without leaving excess waste, which results in weight gain.

The following symptoms indicate the presence of excess toxins in the body: bloating, constipation, indigestion, low energy, fatigue/brain fog, depression, weight gain, chronic pain, infections, allergies, headaches, and gut/digestion problems.

THE BENEFITS OF DETOXIFYING THE BODY INCLUDE:

- Faster, more effortless weight loss
- More energy and overall improved health
- Improved digestion and less constipation, gas, and bloating
- Fewer allergies and allergic responses to foods
- Less mucus and congestion and the clearing up of sniffles and coughs
- Sense of satisfaction, greater vitality, and a desire to choose better foods and develop better eating habits permanently

Detoxifying the body can be accomplished through various detoxification methods, which I discuss in detail below. I would encourage you to pick two or three methods each week to include as part of your overall health and wellness goals.

When you begin detoxifying, you may notice a change for the better in your health and energy levels within a few days; however, for others it may take a few months. Everyone's toxic overload is different, and many factors come into play, such as your health status, weight, metabolism, age, and genetics. Be patient and remain steadfast throughout the process.

I have done each of these detox methods on numerous occasions and perform my personal favorites on a weekly basis. My twenty-one favorite ways to effectively detoxify and cleanse the body are listed below.

1. Acupuncture
2. Alkaline Water
3. Ayurvedic Massage
4. Bikram Yoga
5. Body Brushing
6. Candida Cleanse
7. Castor Oil Packs
8. Chi Machine
9. Coffee Enema
10. Colon Cleansing
11. Colonics
12. Detox Food Pads and Foot Bath
13. Detox Water (Apple Cider Vinegar Detox)
14. Epsom Salt Bath
15. Foods That Detoxify the Body
16. Green Smoothies
17. Heavy Metal Detox
18. Liver Cleansing
19. Parasite Cleanse
20. Physical Activity
21. Sauna

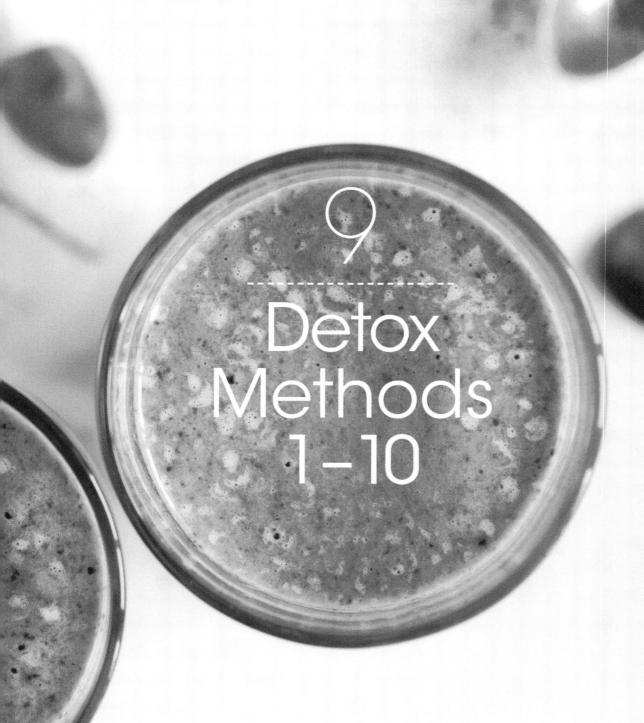

9

Detox
Methods
1 – 10

1. Acupuncture

Acupuncture, a major treatment component of Traditional Chinese Medicine (TCM), is based on balancing Qi (pronounced "chi"), the vital life energy force that nourishes the functions of the body. Through the use of needles, acupuncturists stimulate certain points on the body to alleviate pain or to treat various health conditions. If needles are inserted into these points in the right combinations, the energy flow can be brought back into proper balance to promote healing in the body.

Acupuncture gives the body the tools it needs to restore and heal itself and can be used to detoxify the body and treat chronic pain. If the organs of elimination are open, acupuncture may stimulate the liver, allowing more toxins to be released from the body.

Acupuncture also has a natural diuretic effect. The procedure helps your body detoxify by the elimination of toxins through the urinary tract. It also helps reduce appetite, cravings, and food addictions.

Ease: **Very easy and relaxing (needles are painless)**

Cost: **Varies $75 to $125, per session**

Time: **30 to 40 minutes**

What to Expect: **Reduced appetite or cravings, reduced water weight, and reduced binge eating**

2. Alkaline Water

Your overall pH balance is extremely important to determining good health. The goal is a healthy state of alkalinity because many experts say that disease cannot exist when the body is in an alkaline state. When the body is an acidic state, the body is not healthy. An acidic body puts you at a greater risk for all kinds of disease, chronic illness, and weight gain.

Detoxifying the body makes the body more alkaline. A body that is overloaded with toxins is more prone to becoming acidic. Drinking alkaline water can help to keep the body in an alkaline state. Drinking alkaline water (ion water or hydrogen-rich water) detoxifies the body and leaves the skin looking smoother, more elastic, and more youthful. The benefits of drinking alkaline water are detoxification, better hydration, and increased energy.

Alkaline water has a higher pH level (8 or 9) than regular drinking water (6 or 7). The pH level measures how acidic or alkaline a substance is on a scale of 0 to 14. For example, something with a pH of 1 would be very acidic, and something with a pH of 13 or 14 would be very alkaline. The lower acidity of alkaline water can help neutralize the acid in your body.

A simple way to make your water more alkaline is to add a squeeze of lemon or lime to a glass of distilled water. It's important to use distilled water because tap or bottled water may have additives or artificial ingredients. You can also purchase pH drops and add them to your water as another way to make water more alkaline.

You can buy alkaline water in health food stores or get a portable alkaline water bottle (e.g., IonPod) that converts regular water to alkaline water. A more expensive option is to buy a machine that converts the water from your faucet to alkaline water. An example would be Kangen machine, which costs close to $5,000.

It is recommended that you *not* drink alkaline water with food or within 30 minutes before or after meals. You need to build up how much alkaline water your body can handle, beginning with about 8 ounces a day. If you drink too much alkaline water too quickly, you will get strong detox symptoms, such as headaches or rashes.

Ease: **Easy, just drink up!**

Cost: **Varies, from less than $20 for drops to $5,000 for a machine that converts tap water to alkaline water.**

Time: **None required**

What to Expect: **Detoxification, better hydration, and increased energy**

3. Ayurvedic Massage

Ayurvedic, pronounced "ah-your-vay-dic" massage treats the whole body through touch—physically, mentally, and emotionally. Ayurvedic massage focuses on drawing toxins out of the tissues and into the digestive tract so that they can be eliminated from the body. Lymphatic stimulation with ayurvedic herbal oils help squeeze out toxic accumulation from various channels within the body. Its specialized Dosha oil (warmed), continuous strokes and techniques, full-body steam application, followed by the herbal formula wash/scrub make for an intense, dynamic experience.

Panchakarma, which means "five therapies," is Ayurveda's primary purification and detoxification treatment. It is an expansive cleansing process that releases stored toxins from the body and restores the body's innate healing ability. It is also great at detoxifying the liver and improving the body's ability to metabolize fat. This makes this treatment beneficial for those wanting to detox and lose weight.

There are other Ayurvedic treatments that can address cellulite specifically.

Ease: **Easy and relaxing**

Cost: **$100 to $200, per session**

Time: **1 to 2 hours**

What to Expect: **Stress relief, improved sleep, less cellulite, overall balance**

4. Bikram Yoga

Bikram yoga is one of the most challenging and rewarding detox methods. Bikram Yoga is a form of yoga popularized by Bikram Choudhury in the 1970s in California. The patented practice involves repeating the same twenty-six poses in set cycles in a 90-minute class. I read that doing Bikram yoga for detoxification is one of the best ways to rid your body of unwanted wastes and toxins. Now that I have done Bikram yoga, I would definitely agree! During a Bikram yoga class, the body removes toxic waste through the skin via sweat, as your skin is one of the largest waste-disposal systems in the body.

On its own, yoga is already a powerful fitness regimen because you work out every muscle in the body, making them strong and flexible. The twenty-six Bikram poses are performed in a room temperature of 104°F, with 40 percent humidity. At high temperatures, you will begin to sweat profusely, allowing the toxic waste to be removed from the body. This allows your skin to convert toxins that come from various fats into simpler, more water-soluble compounds that can be easily removed. It has been reported that you actually burn 750 to 900 calories in a 90-minute Bikram yoga session. As an added benefit, you get to learn the techniques of meditation, which can help you relax your mind and alleviate stress. Bikram yoga is an effective means to achieving balance between mind, body, and spirit.

Tips for a Successful Bikram Yoga Session:

- Drink up. If you come to Bikram well-hydrated, you won't need to drink much during the session. Try to drink up to 8 cups of water throughout the day prior to a Bikram session.

- Wear light, breathable clothes. Shorts and tank tops are recommended since you will sweat profusely. Heavy sweats and clothing is not recommended.

- Do not eat 1 to 2 hours before the class. A full stomach may be uncomfortable when you're trying to contract and expand your muscles during the yoga poses. It's best to not eat for at least 1 to 2 hours before the start of the class.

- Arrive 30 minutes prior to class. Give yourself plenty of time to sign up, get dressed, settle in, and get acclimated to the heat.

- Listen to your body. As a first-timer, you're going to be engaging muscles that don't get worked in traditional exercise routines, so you may need to take more breaks than people around you who have been doing it for years. Be kind to yourself and lie down on the mat when you need to and consider it a victory if you manage to stay in the room through the entire class.

Ease: **Very challenging, but rewarding**

Cost: **$10 to $25 per session; cheaper if you buy a monthly package**

Time: **90 minutes**

What to Expect: **Radiant skin, improved flexibility, weight loss, loss of toxins, strengthened immune system, relaxed muscles**

5. Body Brushing

Body brushing (also known as dry brushing) is done with a natural boar-bristle brush, which can be found in health food stores, Whole Foods, or Trader Joe's, or Amazon. Dry brushing on a regular basis lightens the burden on the liver by helping to remove excess waste in the body. Dry brushing stimulates the lymphatic system, which is a secondary circulatory system underneath the skin that rids the body of toxic wastes, bacteria, and dead cells. By body brushing, you move the toxins along and out of the body for elimination. By brushing the body from head to toe with the dry brush—focusing on the lymphatic drainage regions, like behind the knee—you'll improve the efficiency of the whole lymphatic system.

Firm, gentle brush strokes across the skin will improve your blood circulation, clean out clogged pores, and enable your body to remove toxins faster. Body brushing removes dead skin layers and encourages cell renewal for smoother skin. If the liver is the fat-burning organ, then the lymph system can be called a fat-processing system. Cleansing the liver and lymphatic system are key to weight loss.

Further, increasing circulation to the skin could reduce the appearance of cellulite, which is just toxic material accumulated in your body's fat cells.

DIRECTIONS FOR BODY BRUSHING:

1. First remove your clothes and start on dry skin before bathing.
2. Begin brushing the soles of the feet.
3. Next, brush from the ankles to the calves, concentrating on the area behind the knees using long, upward, firm strokes toward the heart. The lymphatic fluid flows through the body toward the heart, so it's important that you brush in the same direction.
4. Your back is the only exception to the rule above; brush from the neck down to the lower back.
5. Then brush from the knees to the groin, the thighs, and the buttocks.
6. If you're a woman, make circular strokes around your thighs and buttocks to help mobilize fat stores, such as cellulite.
7. Then brush the torso, avoiding the breasts.

8. Finally, make long strokes from the wrists to the shoulders and underarms.

9. Never brush over inflamed skin, open sores, sunburned skin, or skin tumors.

10. The entire process should take no more than three to five minutes and will leave your skin feeling totazlly invigorated.

11. Be sure you shower to wash away the dead skin cells and impurities. Then follow with a natural moisturizer of your choice, such as coconut oil.

12. The best times to brush are in the morning before showering or at night before you go to bed.

Ease: **Somewhat easy once you learn the technique**

Cost: **About $10**

Time: **3 to 5 minutes before shower or at bedtime**

What to Expect: **Reduced cellulite, improved circulation, unclogged pores, faster removal of toxins from body.**

6. Candida Cleanse

Candida is a fungus, which is a form of yeast, and a very small amount of it lives in your mouth and intestines. Excess *Candida* in the digestive tract can break down the walls of the intestine and penetrate the bloodstream, releasing toxins into your body and causing leaky gut. This can lead to many different health problems, most commonly fatigue, headache, recurrent yeast infections, and poor memory. Excess *Candida* also causes digestive issues and depression.

HOW TO GET TESTED BY YOUR DOCTOR FOR EXCESS *CANDIDA*:

Stool test: The lab will check for Candida in your colon or lower intestines, and can usually determine the species of yeast by a comprehensive stool test. The stool test is known to be most effective.

Blood test: There are 3 antibodies that should be tested to measure your immune system's response to Candida—IgG, IgA, and IgM. High levels of these antibodies indicate that an overgrowth of Candida is present.

The most important part of treating yeast overgrowth is avoiding sugar and sweets. Additionally, taking antifungal herbs, such as grapefruit seed extract or olive leaf, are helpful, along with repopulating the good bacteria with probiotics.

- -

Ease: **The supplements are easy to take; but it might not be easy to cut down on sweets.**

Cost: **$25 to $50**

Time: **Can require many months to treat**

What to Expect: **More energy, improved mood, better digestion, weight loss, improved concentration**

7. Castor Oil Packs

Castor oil packs are typically used by naturopaths to help stimulate and detoxify the liver. Some find it really helps decongest the liver and minimizes bloating and fluid retention. A castor oil pack is placed directly on the skin to increase circulation and promote elimination and healing of the tissues and organs underneath the skin. It is used to stimulate the liver, relieve pain, increase lymphatic circulation, reduce inflammation, and improve digestion. Castor oil appears to work by drawing blood circulation and biological energy to the area where it is applied and then drawing toxins out of the body.

Castor oil packs are made by soaking a piece of cotton or wool flannel in castor oil and placing it on the abdomen, especially over the liver. The flannel is covered with a sheet of plastic wrap, and a hot water bottle or heating pad is placed over the plastic to heat the pack. You keep the pack on for 30 to 45 minutes while in a relaxed position. Rest while the pack is in place but do not fall asleep and leave the heating pad on all night. After removing the pack, cleanse the area with a solution of water and baking soda. Store the pack in a covered container in the refrigerator. Each pack may be reused up to thirty times. It is generally recommended that a castor oil pack be used for three to seven days in one week as a detoxification treatment. You can also try sleeping with the castor oil pack overnight as well for increased benefit.

You can place the cloth on the right side of the abdomen to stimulate the liver or directly on inflamed and swollen joints and muscle strains. It can be used on the abdomen to relieve constipation and other digestive disorders and on the lower abdomen in cases of menstrual irregularities and uterine and ovarian cysts.

Castor oil should not be taken internally. It should not be applied to broken skin or used during pregnancy, breastfeeding, or during menstrual flow.

Ease: **Somewhat easy, but can be messy**

Cost: **$15 to $30**

Time: **30 to 45 minutes; or can be done overnight**

What to Expect: **Relief from headaches, chronic pain, and dark circles; better lymphatic circulation; reduced inflammation; improved digestion**

8. Chi Machine

The Chi Machine provides a daily detox of the cells by stimulating the lymphatic system, thus improving blood flow. It promotes oxygen flow, energy, and circulation all within 15 minutes.

The Chi Machine is a device that looks like a small suitcase with two ankle rests on the top. You lie on your back on the floor and place your ankles on the rests. The Chi Machine oscillates from right to left, or left to right, approximately 144 times per minute. In just 15 minutes it gives your body the equivalent oxygen benefit of 1½ hours of walking. The figure-8 motion of the machine is similar to the movement of a goldfish. This movement relaxes the nerves and muscles, improves energy flow, and relieves tension in the back, neck, and shoulders. The aerobic activity your body experiences can rejuvenate every aspect of your body while you just lie on the floor with your ankles resting on the machine. It is important to breathe deeply and keep your mind in a peaceful state. It also promotes relaxation and a more restful sleep.

Ease: **Easy and relaxing**

Cost: **$250 to $500**

Time: **10 to 20 minutes**

What to Expect: **Improved circulation, relief from stress, improved metabolic rate, more restful sleep**

9. Coffee Enema

A coffee enema is a therapeutic use of water to wash out the colon and deliver a coffee solution to the body through the rectum. Its effect is very different from drinking coffee. It is used to enhance the elimination of toxins through the liver. More standard enemas use saline solution to cleanse the body, but it is thought by some that the caffeine in coffee provides a more complete cleanse, which is why this is one of my favorite detox methods.

Coffee enemas are powerful detoxifiers due to some alkaloids in the coffee that stimulate the production of glutathione, the master detoxifier in the body. Glutathione helps the body rid itself of dangerous metals such as mercury.

Most colon hydrotherapists can perform coffee enemas right after your colonic. Or you can buy coffee enema kits that let you perform them in the comfort of your home.

- -

Ease: **Can be cumbersome to do at home; easy if done with a colonic**

Cost: **$30 to $60**

Time: **15 minutes to make; 15 minutes to perform when done at home**

What to Expect: **Detoxifies and helps repair the liver; relief from constipation, insomnia, and memory problems; improved digestion; increased energy level; improved mental clarity and mood**

10. Colon-Cleansing Herbs

One way to cleanse the colon is with herbs and supplements, such as powder or capsules. Cleansing the colon with herbs or supplements can help the colon expel its contents. You can find colon-cleansing supplements online, in health food stores, supermarkets, or drugstores. Their primary purpose is to force the colon to expel its contents and draw out old fecal matter.

One of the main theories behind colon cleansing is the belief that undigested foods can cause mucus buildup in the colon. This buildup produces toxins, which enter the blood's circulation, poisoning the body. Thus, colon cleansing will clear toxins from the body or neutralize them and clear out excess mucus and congestion.

A nice benefit of colon cleansing is the reduction of constipation. A poor diet that deprives someone of essential nutrients can cause the intestinal walls to become lined with a plaque-like substance that is not healthy. Colon cleansing not only helps remove the junk from intestinal walls, it also allows waste to pass off more freely. The other noticeable benefit is the elimination of diarrhea, which is normally caused by toxins and can cause problems for the whole process of solidifying the waste.

A very powerful and effective colon cleanser that I've used for overnight results is a magnesium-oxygen supplement. It combines magnesium oxide compounds that have been ozonated and stabilized to release oxygen throughout the entire digestive system over 12 hours or more. The magnesium acts as a vehicle to transport the oxygen throughout the body and has the gentle effect of loosening toxins and acidic waste and transporting them out of the body. Oxygen also supports the growth of friendly bacteria, which is essential for proper digestive and intestinal health.

Magnesium-oxygen supplements are safe for regular use, but I would recommend they be used only periodically during heavy detoxification and cleansing to help keep the colon clean and increase bowel activity. My favorite brand is Mag07, which has been helpful in my personal journey of cleansing and detoxification. This is also a good alternative for my clients who cannot afford or do not have access to colonics (i.e., colon hydrotherapy). Using Mag07, some clients have experienced decreased bloating, gas, and constipation. However, for me, it's knowing that I'm eliminating toxins and waste from my entire digestive tract that provides the biggest benefit.

For intensive colon cleansing, magnesium-oxygen supplements taken for seven to ten days are an effective way to jump-start a detoxification program. They are safe for regular use and can also be used on a longer-term basis for daily, ongoing detoxification. In contrast to synthetic laxatives like senna, a quality magnesium-oxygen supplement is nonhabit-forming and actually strengthens all the organs' functions, making it a safe long-term option.

As always, check with your doctor and be sure to follow the directions on the label. For most people, anywhere from three to five supplements taken at bedtime for seven to ten days will provide an effective colon cleansing. If you experience loose stools or other side effects, simply reduce the dosage and be sure to take just one a day. And please watch the stool to see what comes out. You will be amazed and, possibly, disgusted.

You can also find colon-cleansing products on the Internet or in health food stores, supermarkets, or pharmacies. They include strong herbal teas, enzymes, loose powders, or capsules. My favorite colon-cleansing kit, which involves taking many supplements over a number of days, is by Colonix.

Ease: **Varies. Mag07 is the easiest to take; Colonix requires multiple supplements throughout the day.**

Cost: **Mag07, $15 to $20; Colonix, $50 to $90**

Time: **Mag07, nightly for 7 to 10 days, then 1 to 2 per week for maintenance; Colonix takes about 30 days.**

What to Expect: **Less bloating, gas, and constipation; great for folks who struggle to have a bowel movement every day.**

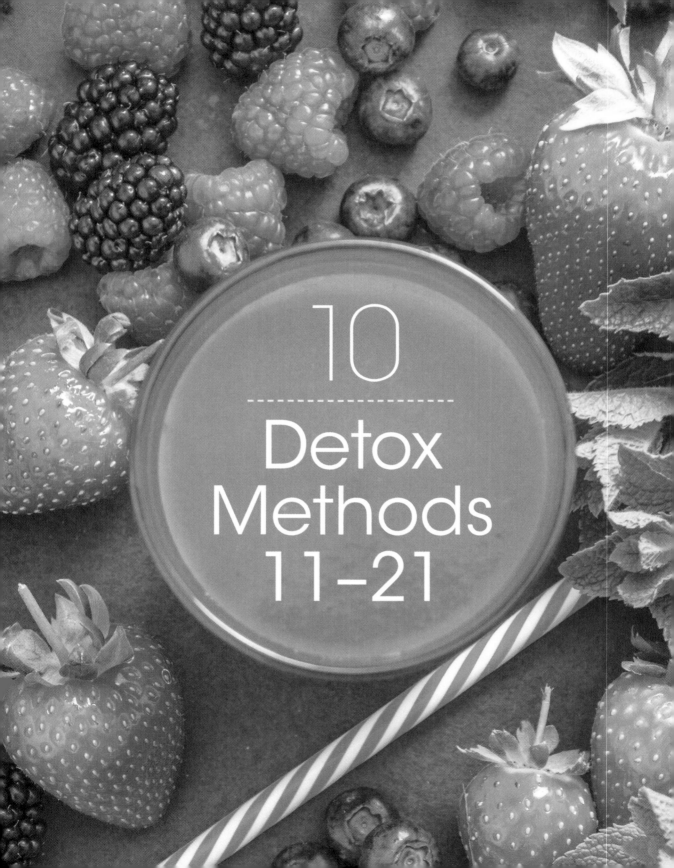

10

Detox
Methods
11–21

11. Colonics

Colonics, also known as colon hydrotherapy or colonic irrigation, is an infusion of water into the rectum by a colon therapist to remove waste and impacted fecal matter from the colon cleanse. Colon hydrotherapy is a gentle washing of the large intestine using purified water. People do colonics to rid their colons of excess toxins that have accumulated over time from the foods they eat, and other environmental toxins, such as pollution, medications, household cleaners, and pesticides.

So what happens during a colonic session? The client lies on a table, and the therapist uses a machine to run water very slowly into the colon. When slight pressure builds up in the colon, the water is released. It can be relaxing after you get started and comfortable. As the water is flowing out through a glass viewing tube, the abdominal area is gently massaged. This process is repeated during the 30- to 45-minute treatment. The therapists may use a variety of water pressures and temperatures. Colonics work somewhat like an enema but involve much more water and none of the odors or discomfort.

One caution about colonics: The colonic will cause your body to get rid of all of its good bacteria along with the bad, but unless you are extremely unhealthy or weak, your body will replenish the good bacteria within twenty-four hours. Nevertheless, you should always take a probiotic supplement after a colonic to replenish the good bacteria right away. A good colon therapist will always provide you with probiotics (good bacteria) at the end of your colonics session.

If you choose to research colonics and decide to include them as part of your detoxification process, you probably want to go at least once a week for up to six weeks, particularly when you first begin aggressively detoxifying the body. That is because you are drawing out toxins, and if they are not eliminated quickly they can cause detox symptoms that become uncomfortable. If your body is managing the toxins and waste well through normal daily bowel movements (one to two per day), then you probably don't need to have a colonic. If your bowel movements are less frequent than once a day, it may be a good idea to do a colonic to get your bowels moving more frequently.

There are no major drawbacks to a properly administered colonic by a trained colon hydrotherapist. You don't need to be concerned about the safety of colonics as long as they're done with a certified colon therapist on a good-quality machine.

Ease: **Relatively easy and relaxing**

Cost: **$60 to $90 per session**

Time: **1 hour**

What to Expect: **Less bloating, gas, and constipation; best for folks who struggle to have a bowel movement every day.**

12. Detox Foot Pads and Foot Bath

DETOX FOOT PADS

This just might be the easier detox method of them all. Detox foot pads are a quick and easy way to rid the body of toxins. They are like large white bandages that have a variety of ingredients and herbs that help the body draw out toxins, even heavy metals and poisons. You put them on the bottoms of your feet overnight, held on by adhesive strips. In the morning, you discard them. They are helpful with aches, pains, sore muscles, joint pains, swelling, and bloating.

Detox foot pads use the same philosophy as acupuncture, as the foot contains more than 60 acupuncture points. When blood circulates through the foot, the detox foot pad utilizes these acupuncture points to draw out toxins. As toxins are pulled from the tissues and cells in the body, they end up in the feet where they can be eliminated with the detox foot pad.

My favorite brand is BodyRelief Foot Pads or Asako Detox Foot Pads, which really helps me with joint aches and pains.

DETOX FOOT BATH

The detox foot bath (ionic foot bath), found in many salons and spas, works by soaking your feet in a warm saltwater solution made up of many different toxin-drawing ingredients. An ionic detox foot bath is a natural method of assisting the body in eliminating harmful toxins and heavy metals. The ionic activity in the water shoots through your body fat and draws the toxins out through the hundreds of pores in your feet. Thirty minutes is the average time for a detox foot bath, which costs a little more than the foot pads ($15 vs. $60 for a detox foot bath). A detox foot bath is said to make joint movement easier in the knees and elbows. It's an alternative medicine option for people who suffer headaches and chronic joint and bone pain.

A detox foot bath is very simple and extremely relaxing. It is typically offered as a spa service under the name of Aqua Chi Foot Bath.

Ease: **Very easy and relaxing**

Cost: **Foot pads, about $15 for 10 foot pads; foot bath, about $60 per session**

Time: **Foot pads (done overnight while sleeping); Foot bath (30 to 45 minutes)**

What to Expect: **Decrease in aches, pains, swelling.**

13. Detox Water (Apple Cider Vinegar Drink)

Drinking apple cider vinegar (ACV) diluted with water one to three times a day is an easy and effective way to detoxify and improve digestion. ACV has great cleansing properties due to its rich content of minerals, vitamins, and enzymes. It helps the body remove toxins and waste more efficiently before they have time to accumulate and damage the body. ACV is known to aid digestion and improve bowel movements. It also helps to detoxify the liver, purify the blood, and improve circulation due to its powerful enzymes that break down bad cholesterol and prevent it from clogging your arteries.

ACV stimulates your metabolism and makes you burn fat faster. Because ACV stimulates digestion, it also reduces the amount of time fats remain in the digestive tract. If fats are present longer than necessary during digestion, more fat will be absorbed by the body.

If you are going to use ACV for weight loss, you need to drink it first thing every morning. You can drink it up to three times per day—before each meal—to accelerate results.

THE RECIPE I LIKE CONSISTS OF THE FOLLOWING:

- 2 tablespoons raw unfiltered apple cider vinegar
- 6 to 8 ounces water
- squeeze of lemon
- dash of cayenne pepper (optional)
- (You can add stevia to taste but it's not necessary.)
- My favorite brand of ACV is Bragg Apple Cider Vinegar.

- -

Ease: **Easy but doesn't taste great**

Cost: **Less than $5**

Time: **2 to 3 minutes to make**

What to Expect: **Benefits include improved digestion, reduced bloating, help with weight loss.**

14. Epsom Salt Bath

Epsom salt is rich in both magnesium and sulfate. Magnesium and sulfate can be easily absorbed through the skin. In an Epsom salt detox bath, the magnesium sulfate is absorbed through the skin, which helps to draw out toxins, extra fluid, and cellular waste from the body. By drawing out the excess fluid in your body, Epsom salt baths help to eliminate bloating and excess water weight. In fact, celebrities often use Epsom salt baths two to three days before a big event so that they look their absolute best.

To make an Epsom salt bath: Start slowly by adding 1 tablespoon of Epsom salt to your bath water. Gradually, over time and several baths, increase the amount of salt to two cups. If you start with big quantities without a gentle introduction first, you might suffer some adverse symptoms, like extreme fatigue. Soak in the bath for 15 to 20 minutes and unwind. Don't stay in the bath for longer than 25 minutes or you might end up exhausting yourself. Be sure to rehydrate well during and after your hot bath. Epsom salt baths can be done once or twice per week.

To provide even more benefit, you can add ten drops of the following essential oils, which will help with various conditions:

- Lavender: calming and relaxation
- Cedarwood: depression and mood swings
- Peppermint: fatigue
- Chamomile and rosemary: headaches

Ease: **Very relaxing**

Cost: **$5 to $10**

Time: **5 minutes to prepare, 20 minutes to soak**

What to Expect: **Detoxification, lower stress, relief of pain and muscle cramps, less bloating and water weight**

15. Foods That Detoxify

When you eat natural, organic, healthy foods, especially raw foods, you keep your insides clean and tend to look radiant despite your age. Detoxification is about cleansing and nourishing the body from the inside out. By eliminating toxins, then feeding your body with healthy nutrients, detoxifying can help you maintain optimum health.

THE FOLLOWING FOODS DO AN IMPRESSIVE JOB OF DETOXIFYING THE BODY:

- *Almonds:* Just a couple of small handfuls a day can help cleanse waste deposits from the body, according to a recent study from the *Journal of the National Cancer Institute.* Almonds are high in fiber, calcium, magnesium, and protein, which help to stabilize blood sugar and remove impurities from the bowels.

- *Beans.* Beans contain the potent enzyme cholecystokinin, which naturally suppresses your appetite while providing protein to your liver to help detox your body. Add them to salads or eat them as a main dish or a side dish.

- *Beets.* Not only can eating beets boost your energy and lower your blood pressure, it can help you fight cancer and boost your brain. Beets contain a unique mixture of natural phytochemicals and minerals that will help you fight infection, purify your blood, and cleanse your liver. When you're detoxing, beets will help by making sure the toxins you're drawing out of your tissues and cells actually make it out of your body via sweat, pooping, or peeing.

- *Broccoli sprouts.* Broccoli sprouts are extremely high in antioxidants and can help stimulate the detoxification enzymes in the digestive tract like no other vegetable. The sprouts are actually more effective than the fully grown vegetable.

- *Citrus fruit.* These fruits, which include grapefruit, lemon, lime, and orange, aid the body in flushing out toxins as well as jump-starting the digestive tract with enzymatic processes. They also aid the liver in its cleansing processes. To increase detoxification, start each morning with a warm glass of lemon water. Vitamin C transforms toxins into digestible material.

- *Garlic.* This pungent bulb stimulates the liver to produce detoxification enzymes that help filter out toxic residues in the digestive system. Adding sliced or cooked garlic to any dish will help aid any detox diet.

- *Green leafy veggies.* Fill your refrigerator with kale, wheatgrass, spinach, spirulina, alfalfa, Swiss chard, arugula, and other organic leafy greens. These veggies work best for cleansing the body when eaten raw or juiced raw in a juicer. These plants will help give a chlorophyll boost to your digestive tract. Chlorophyll rids the body of harmful environmental toxins from smog, heavy metals, herbicides, cleaning products, and pesticides. Green leafy veggies are also high in naturally occurring sulfur and glutathione, which helps the liver eliminate harmful chemicals. One way to add these vegetables to your diet is through drinking green smoothies (see Chapter 2).

- *Omega-3 oils.* Use hemp oil, avocado oil, olive oil, fish oil, or flaxseed oil to lubricate the intestinal walls, allowing the toxins to be absorbed by the oil and eliminated by the body.

- *Onions.* Onions, scallions (green onions), and shallots are sources of sulfur-containing amino acids. According to Patrick Holford and Fiona McDonald Joyce, authors of the book *The 9-Day Liver Detox Diet*, sulfur drives a critical liver-detox pathway known as sulfation. The amino acids present in onions provide the raw materials to make glutathione, a detoxifying compound in the liver. Glutathione detoxifies the body with the acetaminophen and caffeine that pass through the organ. These authors recommend eating a small onion, a shallot, or four green onions raw every day to garner the full detoxifying effect. Raw red onions are particularly beneficial as they contain quercetin, a natural anti-inflammatory that enhances liver function.

- *Seeds and nuts.* Incorporate more of the easily digestible seeds and nuts into your diet. These include flaxseed, pumpkin seeds, almonds, walnuts, hemp seeds, sesame seeds, chia seeds, Siberian cedar nuts, and sunflower seeds.

Ease: **Easy, you just eat**

Cost: **Inexpensive**

Time: **However much time you want to spend on food prep**

What to Expect: **More radiant health, improved digestion, feelings of youthfulness**

16. Green Smoothies

Green smoothies have such a powerful ability to detox the body, they deserve a category all by themselves. Green smoothies give your body the quality nutrition it needs while cleansing your cells and insides. Vitamins, minerals, and other nutrients will be absorbed by your body more efficiently, allowing your cells to become like new as you begin to look and feel younger. Green smoothies are filled with chlorophyll, which is similar in structure to the hemoglobin in human blood. So every time you drink a green smoothie, it's like receiving a blood transfusion. They are a powerful cleansing method for the body.

As I referenced at the beginning of this section, once your body has utilized nutrients from the food you consume, it disposes of the unused food particles and waste produced by the digestive process. If you don't properly and completely eliminate undigested food, whatever remains backs up and leave toxins and waste in your body. But thanks to green smoothies, you can get the fiber you need to cleanse your body, tone your digestive system, and eliminate toxins.

Many people have successfully used the 10-Day Green Smoothie Cleanse, which I've written about in a book by the same title to detox the body and jump-start weight loss!

Ease: **Somewhat easy to make**

Cost: **$10 to $20**

Time: **5 minutes to make**

What to Expect: **Weight loss, increased energy, reduction in food cravings, clearer skin**

17. Heavy Metal Detox

Heavy metals such as mercury, lead, and aluminum can accumulate in the body and trigger health conditions like heart disease, thyroid problems, autism, infertility, and dementia. Other common symptoms include fatigue, memory issues, brain fog, joint pain, and weakness/muscle pain. A heavy metal detox removes heavy metals and other toxic substances from the body and replenishes important nutrients for improved health and well-being.

Before doing a heavy metal detox, you want to get a blood test to assess your total body load of mercury and other heavy metals. A popular treatment is to use DMSA, which is FDA-approved, or other binding agents to pull the mercury out of your body. Your doctor can help you get access to the best method of treatments. Other heavy metal detox supplements include chlorella, cilantro, and milk thistle. Saunas also help with a heavy metal detox.

Ease: **You just take various supplements**

Cost: **Varies because it requires testing to determine the most effective treatment methods**

Time: **Varies; it can take months or even years to remove mercury and other heavy metals from the body**

What to Expect: **Reduction of or complete disappearance of symptoms related to toxins and heavy metals; increased energy; improved sleep patterns; elimination or reduction of stomach problems, muscle aches, and joint pain.**

18. Liver Cleansing

The liver, nicknamed the fat-burning organ, is key to detoxing and fat burning in the body. Although there are several organs of elimination in the body, most health practitioners will agree that the liver is the primary one. It has been said that the length and quality of life depends on proper liver function. The liver works day and night to cleanse the blood of toxins such as chemicals, bad bacteria, and other foreign substances. The liver is also responsible for breaking down fats in the body. It is critical to keep the liver clean and healthy and working at peak performance.

One easy way to cleanse the liver is to take herbs/supplements such as milk thistle, dandelion root, and burdock. These herbs are all-natural and very effective. You'll find that many products on the market combine these herbs into one supplement so that you can achieve the best results. As you look for products to help you cleanse your liver, be sure to use only those that are all-natural and gentle on the body. My favorite two liver-cleansing supplements are Liver Rescue by HealthForce and Livatone Plus by Dr. Sandra Cabot.

Additionally, an inexpensive option is to drink 2 tablespoons of raw and unfiltered apple cider vinegar in 8 ounces of water every morning and night. (See "Apple Cider Vinegar" in Appendix A.) Do this for a few weeks to a few months until fat burning increases in the body. Additionally, you may notice that the symptoms of a sluggish liver improve. Symptoms of a sluggish liver include:

- Eyes are no longer white
- Poor skin tone, including acne or break-outs around the nose, cheeks, and chin
- Dark circles under eyes
- Yellow-coated tongue
- Bitter taste in the mouth
- Headaches
- Moodiness and irritability

A liver cleanse can be a rejuvenating experience that yields numerous health benefits.

Ease: **Easy, you just take supplements or drink apple cider vinegar in water**

Cost: **$5 to $40 for supplements**

Time: **Almost none**

What to Expect: **Reduction in dark circles under eyes, improved skin tone, brightening of whites of eyes, boost in metabolism and thus fat burning.**

19. Parasite Cleanse

Because parasites can live in the stomach and intestines, they suck up nutrients from your body, preventing you from getting the nourishment you need from your food. They can cause great damage, weakening the immune system and causing disease.

Some of the most common parasites—such as roundworms, tapeworms, pinworms, and blood flukes—can cause abdominal cramping, bloating, foul gas, belching, and other chronic digestive issues. Symptoms include depression, anxiety, body aches, headaches, eye aches, sometimes anal itching.

THE TWO MOST COMMON RED FLAGS THAT INDICATE YOU MAY HAVE PARASITES ARE:

- chronic digestive issues, including constipation, diarrhea, bloating, and gas.
- mental distress, including depression, panic attacks, and anxiety

You only need a parasite cleanse if your doctor confirms that you have parasites, usually found in a comprehensive stool exam. Herbal supplements are a great way to rid the body of parasites. Cloves, wormwood, and black walnut are the herbs to use to get rid of parasites. A parasite cleanse is recommended one or two times per year if symptoms exist.

Ease: **Very easy to take supplements**

Cost: **$25 to $100 for supplements.**

Time: **To rid the body of parasites could take 1 to 3 months**

What to Expect: **Benefits include successful removal of parasites from the digestive tract, which results in less bloating and gut issues, clearer thinking, and increased energy.**

20. Physical Activity

It's important to Get Moving! Physical activity is good for detoxing because it gets the body moving, heart pumping, and lungs breathing deeply. This oxygenates the body to protect it against toxic overload, washing out sludge that accumulates in arteries. Physical activity also helps the organs of elimination function optimally simply by helping to circulate both blood and lymph, enabling the liver and lymph nodes to do the job of cleansing and purifying the blood and lymph, the body's collector of toxic waste.

Physical activity also helps to detoxify the body by reducing the body's subcutaneous fatty tissue. Toxins get stored in fatty tissue, and physical activity will help the body release them.

With physical activity, you breathe deeply with your lungs, bringing oxygen through the blood to the brain and muscles. The lungs increase their capacity as the heart muscle grows stronger, giving off carbon dioxide as a waste product.

As little as 30 minutes of brisk walking can prompt this type of cleansing. Try to move at a pace at which you can breathe evenly yet still carry on a conversation.

Ease: **Somewhat easy (depends on whether you like to move around)**

Cost: **None**

Time: **30 minutes**

What to Expect: **Better circulation and mobility, heart health**

21. Sauna

A sauna session helps you sweat out toxins, burn calories, and come out with glowing skin. It also boosts the immune system and relaxes the muscles. So many benefits!

The skin is the largest organ of elimination for the body. Perspiring through the skin flushes out toxins and impurities. Additionally, the heat of the sauna causes the body's temperature to rise, which can help kill any virus, bacteria, fungus, or parasite in the body.

A sauna session can do more to clean, detoxify, and simply freshen your skin than anything else. The heat from the sauna opens up the pores of the skin, allowing impurities and toxins to flush themselves out of the body. It hydrates and moisturizes the skin and is particularly beneficial to people with dry skin. One of my clients found that by sweating out her toxins in the sauna, her acne cleared up.

A sauna session will speed up metabolism, which in turn results in weight loss. You can burn 300 to 500 calories in 15 to 20 minutes in a sauna, equivalent to one to two hours of brisk walking or one hour of aerobic exercise.

The high temperature of the sauna causes an artificial fever, which sends a "wake-up call" to the immune system and increases the white blood cell count.

The heat also warms and relaxes tense muscles. This relaxation helps to reduce stress levels, revive mental clarity, and improve overall physical and emotional health.

The best type of sauna is an infrared sauna, which produces what is known as radiant heat. The heat of an infrared sauna also penetrates more deeply without the discomfort and draining effect often experienced in a conventional steam sauna. An infrared sauna produces two to three times more sweat volume, and due to the lower temperatures used (110° to 130°F), it is considered a safer alternative for those at cardiovascular risk. It accelerates the removal of toxic wastes lodged in the fatty tissues. The sweating caused by deep heat helps eliminate dead skin cells and improve skin tone and elasticity. The heat produced in infrared saunas is extremely helpful for various skin conditions, including acne, eczema, and cellulite. Plus studies have shown that you can burn 600 calories in 30 minutes in an infrared sauna.

I enjoy sitting in the sauna several times a week because it has both health benefits and beauty benefits.

CAUTIONS:

- The sauna can be dehydrating, so it is important to drink lots of water before and after your session.

- If you have heart issues, particularly sensitive skin or asthma, or if you are pregnant, you should check with your doctor before you sit in a sauna.

Ease: Not too easy; can be hot, so stay hydrated

Cost: About $60 per session at a spa or free at some gyms; $200 for portable sauna; up to $3,000 for wood sauna

Time: 20 to 30 minutes per session; once or twice a week is ideal

What to Expect: Detoxification, weight loss, radiant skin, strengthened immune system, relaxed muscles

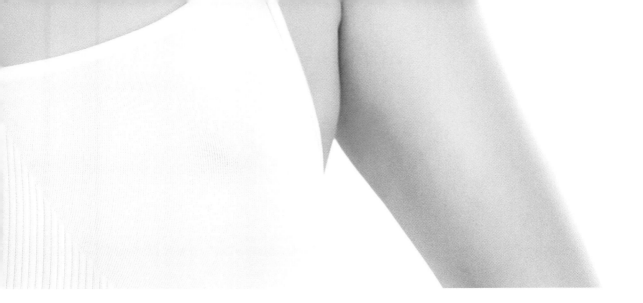

PART 3

SUCCESS STORIES

This section offers a little extra motivation with several success stories from individuals who have experienced the power of green smoothies to increase their energy, change their eating habits, and transform their bodies. People just like you have had extraordinary success. Their stories will help you see that you can have success, too. These individuals have turned back the hands of time, lost 40 or more pounds or have gotten to their goal weight and kept the weight off by incorporating green smoothies and healthy, clean meals into their regimen.

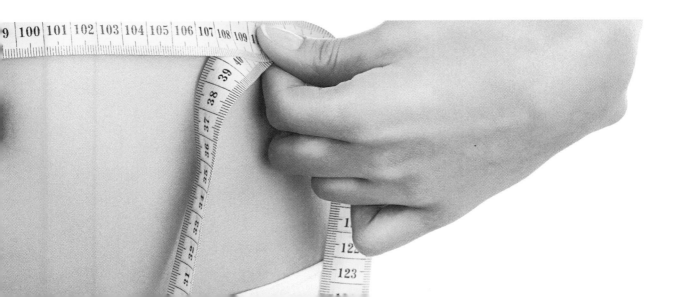

Tammi lost 61 pounds and says, "You are worthy!"

"Starting a new journey is never easy, and staying committed to something is just as hard. Looking in a mirror and not loving the image staring back at you, being disappointed because you can't dress the way you would like, or hearing people say, "You've let yourself go," are enough to put you on guard. The power of a made-up mind is what causes you to take action. I finally decided that I am in control of what happens to me no matter what anybody says or even what I feel. I realized that nothing will change if my mindset isn't right.

"In June, I decided enough was enough. I didn't have any medical issues confronting me, but my family has a history of high blood pressure and diabetes. I didn't want to invite those ailments. My first 10 days of the 10-Day Green Smoothie Cleanse, I remember making my smoothies and packing them in a cooler as we traveled to Memphis with our children's choir. I committed to those 10 days. I gained so much energy that I began to walk daily for at least 30 minutes. The inches were falling off, and I was picking up steam. As I continued incorporating green smoothies into my lifestyle, I've gone from 225 to 164 pounds. I have worn some size 6s, down from 16/18. My shoe size has even shrunk a half size!

"People are looking to me for motivation (not my intended goal). My desire is to help all I can, directly or indirectly. The way I see it, 'As each has received a gift, use it to serve one another, as good stewards of God's varied grace (1 Peter 4:10).' God has allowed so many positive influences in my life since starting this journey that I feel if I ever give up, I'm denouncing his gifts to them and to me, so I keep pressing. I know that this movement is of God.

"If there was one thing I could say to help or to motivate someone, I would say, "You are enough, you are worthy, you will succeed, you have the power to become anything that you set your mind to." It has to become your daily mantra, your pep talk. You have to not only *talk* about it, you have to *be* about it.

160

"Now that I am at my goal weight, I live the DHEMM Life (Detox, Hormonal Balance, Eat Clean, Mental Mastery, Move, see page 198) life. I normally have at least one smoothie per day. I will continue to use Green Smoothies for Life. I've changed my eating habits and also those of my children. I'm known as the girl who is always walking. I'm not done working on me, but I am on the right road finally and for that I am forever grateful.

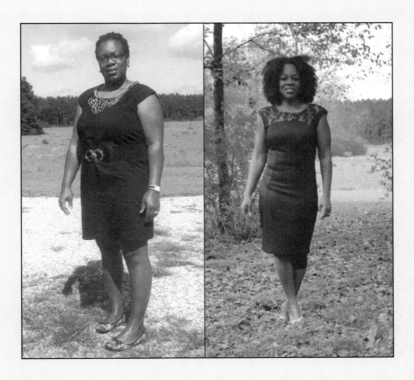

Chelsea lost 40 pounds and got rid of the baby weight!

" When I got pregnant, I used it as an excuse to eat anything and everything in sight, because I was convinced the weight would just fall right off after my son was born. Consequently, I gained over 50 pounds. Nine months after his birth in February, I was only down 15 pounds from the day that I delivered him. My back and ankles ached with the excess weight I was carrying. My skin was always oily and breaking out in acne. My hair was falling out in clumps every time I showered or brushed it. I felt anxious and worried and distracted. Worst of all, I hated the way I felt in my own skin. I never felt comfortable, and I wore girdles and baggy clothes to try and hide my protruding stomach.

"The sadness and depression that I felt fueled me to seek comfort in food. Fried food. Pizza. Cheese. Bread. Beer. I was caught in this vicious cycle. I spent hours a week online researching various 'quick weight-loss' products and spent countless amounts of money on girdles, pills, 'fat burners,' shakes, wraps, workout DVDs, and even hypnosis CDs, and nothing worked. In one final attempt, I typed in 'weight loss' on Amazon .com and found JJ's book *The 10-Day Green Smoothie Cleanse*. I read review after review of people providing testimony to the amazing results they received. I ordered the book and started the following Monday.

"The first few days were rough without coffee, bread, and late-night sweet snacks. I was grumpy, had bad headaches, and everything felt fuzzy. But I just kept pushing through and finally made it to Day 10. For the first time in a very long time, I felt proud of myself. I had stuck with it for 10 days. I didn't buy the success somewhere. I didn't take some 'magic pill' I didn't pay someone to do it for me. I did it myself. All me.

"I hopped on the scale the morning of Day 10 and saw that I had lost an incredible 8 pounds! My skin looked clear and bright. My stomach didn't stick out as far. I had so much more energy. My mental clarity and focus at work were profound. I can't remember the last time I felt so good! This jump start on weight loss was just the thing I needed to continue my journey. I have since continued drinking green smoothies for life, and have even taken up running again—something I loved to do years and years ago. I've lost a total of 40 pounds by incorporating green smoothies into my lifestyle, and I am not stopping anytime soon!"

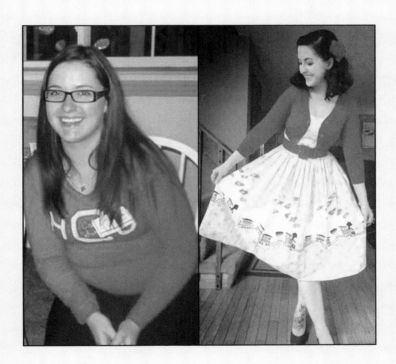

Lisa lost 60 pounds and realized that eating is the key to losing weight.

" For as long as I can remember, I have always been a heavy girl. I never knew what it was like to be thin nor have I ever felt good about my appearance. My self-esteem was at its lowest. I yearned for the approval of others and never really loved myself. This pattern of self-destruction was carried on for over forty-four years.

"On July 20, I came across a Facebook post by a member of the Green Smoothie Cleanse (GSC) Facebook Group. I researched the program and read the many testimonials that were provided, saw their results in the pictures that were posted, and began thinking this could be the answer to my prayer. You see, I had tried several other weight-loss programs and was somewhat successful but was not able to maintain and keep it off. As I continued to read and see all of the positive results, I finally decided to give it a try. All that was required was 10 days, 10 days to a better and healthier me.

"On August 2, I began the 10-Day Green Smoothie Cleanse. It was on this day that my life began changing for the better. I decided to take action and responsibility for what food I eat to fuel my body. No longer do I live to eat, I now eat to live. The first time that I did the Full Cleanse, I successfully completed it and released 12 pounds. From there on, I was rocking and rolling. I have followed JJ's 30-Day Program and now I drink green smoothies for life and have made it a lifestyle for me.

"Since then, I have gained so much more than releasing the pounds. For me it is no longer about the weight loss. Letting go of the pounds is a plus; however, the greatest benefit of this journey has been gaining my confidence and learning how to love myself. I now have a greater appreciation and understanding of how important it is to take care of the temple that God has entrusted me with. Eating is the key to losing, but how you prepare your food and what you choose to eat is more important.

"My kids are my motivation to continue this healthy lifestyle. I have two active young men who are the joy of my life. My desire is to live a long and healthy life and to see them grow up to be strong, healthy, successful men. I realized that if I continued living the path that I was on, it was bound to end earlier than necessary. Seeing the many victories and rewards there are to this lifestyle is also a motivation for me to continue. I continue this lifestyle because it has given me the desire to do better and to strive for greatness.

"Just to name a few of the non-scale victories that I have experienced on this journey:

I discontinued my blood pressure medication after less than 6 months of doing GSC.

I am able to cross my legs.

My skin is now smoother and clearer. No longer do I have problematic dark skin blotches.

I no longer have a double chin.

To date I have released a total of 60 pounds.

"Although, I am a work in progress, I have also learned that this process is not about perfection, instead it is about progress. I may not be perfect, but I am far from where I started. I am a brand-new creature in Christ. I am learning how to speak life into my path. I continue to encourage myself and try to live life as an example to others. I am forty-five years old and feel better and look younger than I have felt in years.

"If there was only one thing that I could tell someone to encourage them to continue on this healthy weight-loss journey, it would be to believe in yourself, know that you are worth it. For this journey is a total transformation process. Not only will it heal the body, it will also heal the mind. Changing your eating habits changes your outlook on life. I finally can truly say I now believe in me, I am stronger, and I am worth all that God has for me. Connect with your inner spirit. Take this journey to greater heights. Never allow anyone to deter you from achieving your goals. Pave the path and tread it with sheer determination. And never give up on you!

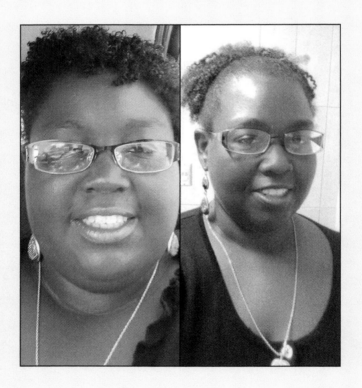

Avicia lost 80 pounds and says, "Everything you need to be successful on this journey is already inside of you!"

"On April 21, 2014, I took the first step toward gaining control of my life by starting the 10-Day Green Smoothie Cleanse (GSC). I had struggled with my weight tremendously in the years and months leading up to that day. I had tried several quick fixes and even spent a few thousand dollars on a personal trainer, but I did not see my desired results. My weight fluctuated over the years, and at my heaviest of 263 pounds at 5'3", I was on the verge of a number of health issues. So, after being tired of talking about it year after year, I took some time to pray and get my mind right, and then I decided to give myself 10 days. My life and health were worth it.

"During the 10 days, I experienced multiple detox symptoms, and by Day 5 I was ready to give up. I remember sitting in my car crying on that day. I was so frustrated with myself and my addiction to food, which had me on such an edge. I wasn't hungry because the smoothies and snacks were very filling, but I hungered for the things that I was trying to break myself free of. Nevertheless, I didn't give up. I kept going. Although it was very challenging, I completed the GSC and lost 9 pounds, gained energy, improved my skin, and gained confidence in myself. It was the most rewarding 10 days of my life, and after that moment I never looked back.

"I continued with JJ's 30-Day Program and continued drinking green smoothies for life. In December I joined the VIP (see Appendix B), group and that opened a whole new door to my weight-loss journey. I learned so much from the group, and I've lost over 80 pounds and kept it off because of it. The VIP group taught me not to fixate on the smoothies, and it has introduced me to many other methods that have helped me maintain my weight loss. Over the past fifteen years, I suffered from severe migraines, which I would get at least eight times a year. Now, those migraines occur only about twice a year. I would get sick as the seasons changed, but since joining the VIP group and utilizing the tools that JJ equips me with, my overall health has improved, and my energy level is higher than it has ever been. I completed my first 8k in March, and that was a very rewarding experience. This is the first time in my life that I actually feel good about who I am.

"The thing that keeps me inspired and motivated to continue on this journey is knowing how far I've come. It took me a long time to see the difference. I would always get compliments from people and that felt great, but it didn't change how I saw myself. I would look at my 'before' and 'after' pictures and see the difference, but when I looked in the mirror I would still see the 263-pound version of me. After attending JJ's Sexy By Summer conference, becoming a certified GSC leader, and meeting so many amazing women on this journey, I have finally learned how to really see me, the version of me that was in the mirror. I had to train my brain to look at me and see what was really there. And for the first time, in July, I looked in the mirror and saw a 175-pound woman looking back at me. I instantly fell in love with her. The hard work, the dedication, the tears, the ups and the downs made me the woman that I am proud to be.

"I maintain my focused mindset by planning out my week. Meal prep is very important for me, and Sundays are typically my prepping days. Since I drink green smoothies for life, I take the time to pre-pack my smoothie ingredients and snacks for the week. I make sure I have everything I need so that I am able to make smart decisions. I like to cook my meals and have them ready to go. For me, this leaves little room for error. I also keep my motivation board visible at all times. I place quotes and pictures that inspire me. I set goals for the week and write them down in my journal. It really helps to keep my thoughts and plans written down.

"If there was one thing I could say to someone to inspire them to continue on this journey, it would be: Know your worth and know that everything you need to be successful on this journey is already inside of you. "

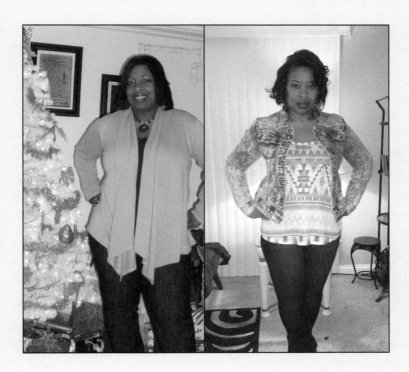

Pamela lost 101 pounds and says, "I have nine people who inspire me, and they all call me Grandma!"

My journey actually started by accident. My son had a green smoothie in his hand, and I asked him, "What is that nasty stuff?" He said, "Try it." After much prodding, I did and found it was surprisingly quite tasty. Then he went on to tell me how he had lost 10 pounds on JJ Smith's 10-Day Green Smoothie Cleanse. The rest, as they say, is history. I started my first Full Cleanse in March. I lost 12 pounds and was so amazed. I continued drinking green smoothies as a part of my lifestyle.

"I had high blood pressure and was morbidly obese. My highest weight was 280 pounds, and I lost 101 pounds! With JJ's 30-Day Program, which always incorporates green smoothies every day, I have been able to do things I never imagined I could do, like zip-lining and riding a bike.

"I had a knee replacement five years ago, and my other knee was always in pain. Now with the weight loss, I don't suffer from knee pain. My blood pressure is normal. I can climb a flight of stairs without being winded. My life has become active.

"I have nine people who inspire me, and they all call me Grandma. I want to be around to watch them grow up and be able to run around with them. I have people tell me that I inspire them to want to lose weight.

"Smoothie and meal prep, bagging the ingredients, and creating a menu for the week help keep me on track. Doing the prep has become part of my weekly routine for the past year. Having my supplements available on my nightstand with a bottle of water reminds me to take them.

"I thought I was destined to be heavy for the rest of my life because no other weight-loss program ever worked for me.

"Remember, you deserve to be healthy!

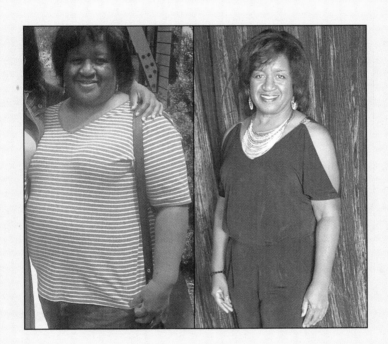

Dorelle lost 60 pounds and says, "Just keep going!"

My journey all started with my feeling very emotional and tired of being called the 'fatso' of the family. I have been above 200 pounds ever since having my four children. Living in Hawaii on a laid-back and relaxed island in the middle of the Pacific Ocean, and loving my starches, I found even more pounds just added on.

"Then I became sick and tired of being sick and tired, literally! Aside from my own issues, my mom suffered a massive heart attack in September, which pushed me even more to change my lifestyle. The night of November 21, I started out by just surfing the net trying to look for a smoothie detox. I know it was all God because He directed me to JJ's 10-Day Green Smoothie Cleanse. The door opened when JJ posted a 10-Day Green Smoothie Challenge on the 10-Day Green Smoothie Facebook page! I said, 'Yes, I will give it a try.' Between December 2014 and September 30, 2015, I have followed JJ's 30-Day Program and continue to incorporate green smoothies into my daily regimen and have lost a total of 60 pounds, and I am still going. Though I'm not where I want to be just yet, I'm surely not where I used to be. I suffered from really bad sciatica on the left side. After drinking green smoothies, I started heading for the gym and jumping on the elliptical. Even if I had pain, I would push through. Within weeks, the pain started to decrease. And now, thank you Jesus, I have no pain! My hubby suffered a heart attack on December 25, which helped me to stay focused on my lifestyle changes.

"I joined JJ's Private VIP Group (see Appendix B) and have been glued to the motivation from everyone! I am truly inspired by the results. They are real, and it works. I'm determined and focused on the prize. I love and look forward to making my smoothies daily.

"My advice is to seek God for the strength, be in the Word, because ultimately He gives us strength and guidance. Don't give up. It's important to remember how we used to be very unhealthy and unhappy, to look at the before and after pictures, and look for inspiration daily. This has been the most rewarding lifestyle change that works. My lifestyle changed because I so wanted it to.

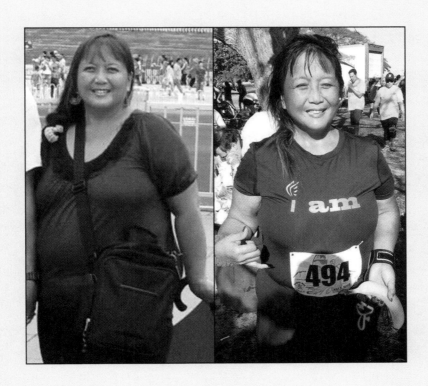

Sabrina who lost 74 pounds, says, "Trust God and imagine tomorrow happier and healthier than today!"

" The journey to improve my health started in December. When I was diagnosed with rheumatoid arthritis in May 2012, my life completely changed. I went from working 80 hours per week to not being able to work at all. I felt like a failure. I weighed 268 pounds and felt ashamed and disappointed in myself. People said cruel things to me because of my weight. I even lost friends because I was not able to participate in the numerous activities they would plan.

"The day I read Meka Taft's story on the Green Smoothie Cleanse Facebook support page, my thought process changed. The tips she gave and her overall health improvement made me realize I had nothing to lose. If the doctors had been trying different medications on me for 18 months, then I could definitely give this a try the correct way for 10 days. I didn't tell my family what I was doing. I just surprised them after my first Full Green Smoothie Cleanse and continued drinking green smoothies month after month, following JJ's 30-Day Program as well. When I showed up at our annual Christmas gathering, I was already 20 pounds lighter and carrying a smoothie. I felt excited, confident, and, best of all, I was walking without pain. My family was so happy for me.

"As of today, I have lost 74 pounds. I went from wearing a tight size 20 (2X–3X), to a comfortable size 12. The other day I even wore size 10 pants! The excitement that I feel from just trying on my old clothes each week brings tears to my eyes.

"The blessings have continued. My health has improved tremendously. I no longer take medication for diabetes and high blood pressure or the steroids to control my RA flare-ups. My RA injections have now been moved to every other week instead of weekly. I'm walking, running, and feeling stronger every day. My doctors are amazed at my improvement and will be making a decision for me to return to work soon.

"The mind-set that keeps me going is to think, 'If I eat this now, how will I look or feel tomorrow?' I think of how wonderful I felt when I was chosen to walk the red carpet at JJ's Sexy by Summer Conference. Most important, I am proud to see the way my son looks at me today. His eyes used to be filled with pain as he witnessed the pain his mom was in every day. He knew he could do nothing to help me. Today, I am a better living example for my son. I never leave home without a lunch packed, no matter how short my travel is. I now know how to read labels on food items and make healthier choices. I still continue to motivate myself by keeping old pictures of myself posted around my home.

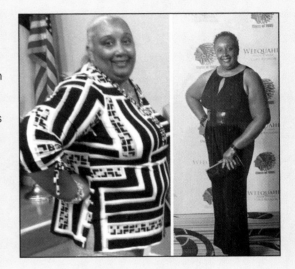

"As of today, I have eight family members I help daily with their own health and green smoothie journey. Motivating them also keeps me motivated because I won't give any advice without doing the same work myself. I've always been the go-to person in my circle of family and friends. Having others choose to come to me for help or advice really warms my heart.

"I never imagined that healing would be in the form of a nutritionist. I was looking for that miracle drug or mistaken diagnosis. It turned out that JJ Smith is the person God placed in my life! And those green smoothies are my new miracle drugs! My one piece of advice to others in a similar situation would be: Trust God and imagine tomorrow happier and healthier than today!

Melanie lost 58 pounds and says, "I love the way my husband looks at me!"

It was January when I made my mind up to do something about my weight. It had come to a point where I didn't recognize the person staring back at me in the mirror. I did not realize how large I'd become. I guess I figured as long as my husband was happy, I was happy, though I truly wasn't and needed to change for me.

"On several different occasions, my doctor had given me handouts for a 1,600-calorie diet and a walking exercise. I'd always glanced at it and throw it away. My blood pressure was consistently around 135/110 or higher. My triglyceride number (bad cholesterol) was 248 and the acceptable range is 35 to 165. I always felt fatigued, tired, and lazy. I could barely walk up a flight of stairs without being tired and out of breath.

"I had my bestie in one ear inviting me to walk or work out with her, and I had my cousin in the other ear telling me about *The 10-Day Green Smoothie Cleanse*. I finally made the commitment to join my bestie in January, for our first 10-Day Cleanse. I was skeptical in the beginning that this would actually work for me. But I made the commitment to finish it.

"I weighed 258 pounds prior to my first cleanse, the heaviest I'd ever been. I was wearing sizes ranging from 20 to 22 and 2X to 3X and was about to purchase a size 24. That is when I said, "No, no more. I cannot go up another size." That was it for me.

"I lost 10 pounds after completing the first cleanse and was hooked from that point on. I continued with JJ's 30-Day Program and have continued drinking green smoothies each month. I was committed to this lifestyle for quite some time, having two smoothies daily, approved snacks, and a lean meal. I wanted to learn more, so I eventually purchased JJ's other book, *6 Ways to Lose Belly Fat*

Without Exercise. I wanted to know everything that JJ Smith knew. I try to apply everything that I know will help me on this journey. I know what I've read will help me because there are too many testimonies of success and I'm now a success story.

"I now drink green smoothies for life and have lost a total of 58 pounds, weighing in at 200. I'm 10 pounds away from my first goal and 25 pounds away from my next one. I now wear a size 14, not a 14W. This is awesome! My blood pressure stays within the normal range, a near perfect 122/80. My triglycerides are at a normal 71, down from 248. Awesome! I'm fully energized and have mental clarity now. I exercise five or six days weekly, sometimes multiple times a day.

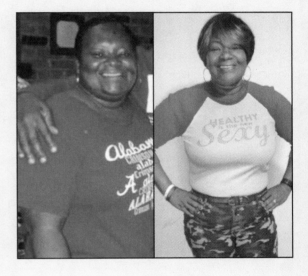

"My motivation comes from various things: I like not feeling tired. I like the person who is staring back at me in the mirror. I like having overall better health. I like being a motivator to others. I love the way my husband looks at me. I'm my biggest motivator. I look at old pics often to remind myself of where I don't want to go back to. I now eat to be healthy.

"I would tell anyone on this journey to embrace all of your NSV (non-scale victories). Those, too, are a part of your journey and should not be discounted. Your weight will fluctuate on this journey. Stay the course by detoxing your body, eating clean, and exercising. Stay focused on your goals and don't get sidetracked by the obstacles (scale), and you will be unstoppable at reaching your goal and being healthy."

Carol lost 35 pounds and says, "I learned the correct way to care for myself!"

On April 10, I started the 10-Day Green Smoothie Cleanse. My weight was the highest it had been in years. The first few days were difficult. I am sure I was not the only person struggling. I remember reading "It's Mind Over Matter." During the Cleanse, the Facebook page was such a great support to me. In addition, anytime I had a question, JJ would answer it.

"On Day 4, I knew I was going to finish strong. During the 10 days, I had no cravings for the foods I used to enjoy. I had so much energy (I didn't even have to exercise a lot) and slept like a baby at night. Come Day 10, I felt like a new person. Weighing in the following morning, I had lost 10 pounds as well as the inches. I was wearing clothes that I hadn't worn in a long time.

"I currently have been following the green smoothies for life plan for 18 months and, as a VIP Member (see Appendix B), I have lost 35 pounds during my journey and have learned how to maintain it. I joined the VIP group to broaden my knowledge. I also was selected to be an Ambassador to help guide others. The VIP group consists of a lot of amazing people from all around the world. It's incredibly inspiring to read about and see pics on Facebook that show how people have changed their lives. It keeps you pushing to do better for yourself. If you post a question, they will respond to you with the correct way of doing things. We have the best support group.

"As far as my health goes, I can honestly say I feel the best I have in a very long time. I have more energy. I used to take Tylenol almost daily for headaches or just to sleep at night. In the last 18 months of drinking green smoothies, I have taken Tylenol only one time. All my doctors say to me, 'Whatever you are doing, keep it up.'

"I highly recommend that anyone who is looking for a change in their life regarding weight and overall health join this wonderful green smoothie family and community."

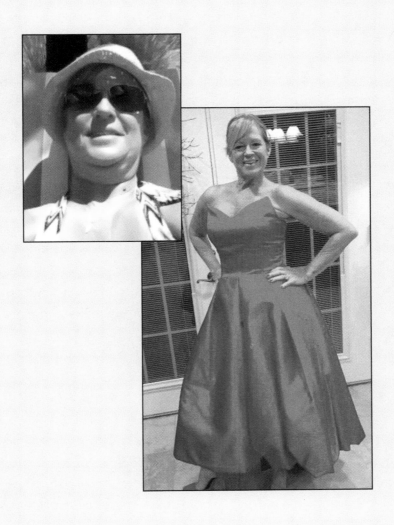

Sharen lost 82 pounds and says, "Enjoy the journey!"

" On this lifestyle change I call my 'extraordinary journey,' I have lost a total of 82 pounds. Prior to starting this green smoothie journey, I weighed 276. I was diagnosed with hypothyroidism (total thyroidectomy 2013), insulin resistance, and the beginning signs and symptoms of osteoarthritis. Throughout the course of my unhealthy lifestyle, I attempted many diets: Weight Watchers, low-carb, and Plexus Slim, just to name the more popular ones. I was able to lose weight with all of them; however, I always later regained it, plus more.

"In October, I started reading about the health benefits of drinking infused water and light exercise. I came across a young lady whose body had been transformed by her weight loss, and I wanted to follow whatever she did to not only lose so much weight but to also look healthy and young at the same time. I was so surprised that she had not had surgery or liposuction. It was at this point I was introduced to JJ Smith! By the end of October, I had started my first Full Green Smoothie Cleanse and lost 13.5 pounds, and by following JJ's 30-Day Program and continuing with my green smoothies, I am down 82 pounds.

"I have been so blessed and am extremely thankful for staying connected with the JJ's Facebook groups. This has kept me motivated and inspired me to stay focused on this journey. Even on the days I have a 'cheat meal,' I am not hard on myself or even feel that I have to 'start over.' I am learning to redirect my lifestyle to what I have become comfortable with doing, which is drinking at least one to two smoothies a day, eating nutritious clean meals, choosing healthy snacks, and using other detox methods to facilitate weight loss. This program provides me with a sense of 'wholeness' that I have not been able to experience before.

"It's funny, sometimes when I walk past someone I haven't seen in a while, either they don't recognize me or they may give a double look and say 'Sharen?' It really makes me feel good and gives me a great sense of accomplishment. I have been able to encourage some of my family and friends to join me in this journey. Some have done very well and some have not. For those of us who have been able to own this journey, it's been extraordinary.

"The one thing I would say as encouragement would be, 'Enjoy the journey!'

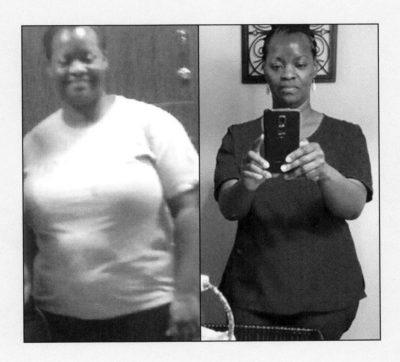

Dorissa lost 55 pounds and says, "Commit to victory, no quitting allowed!"

" I have a 'servant's heart.' That's just the way God 'wired' me. I get joy from serving others, be it my eighty-four-year-old mother, who is experiencing the final stages of Alzheimer's (hospice); or my daughter, who was born mentally and physically challenged; or the homeless family on the street. Serving is what I was born to do.

"I started this green smoothie journey (with my hubby) a week after our birthdays, on March 27, because I wanted to live in my God-given purpose, and in order to do that, I realized I needed to be healthy and fit—mentally, spiritually, and physically. I realized that I can't give my best, if I'm not at my best.

"I can't give if I'm depressed.

"I can't serve and help others if I'm tired.

"I can't find solutions if I can't think.

"I can't move if I'm feeling lethargic.

"I thank God for the blessed day I learned about JJ Smith and the 10-Day Green Smoothie Cleanse. I followed it to a T, never, *almost*, never deviating from the recipes or approved snacks. Since my journey began, I have completed JJ's 30-Day Program and continue to drink green smoothies for life.

"I used to suffer from high blood pressure, insulin resistance, estrogen dominance, hypothyroidism, brain fog, constant fatigue during the day, sleepless nights, shortness of breath, skin rashes, and lupus symptoms (aches and pains). But not anymore. To date, I have lost an amazing grand total of 55 pounds! Since I've had my hormones checked (per the DEHMM system, see page 197), I expect to lose even more!

"I am inspired and motivated each day by God's reminder that every day is a gift. Every day is another opportunity to 'get it right.' Every day is one day closer to everything working out for my good (Romans 8:28). That means the good, the bad, and the downright difficult, unfair, unjust, and ugly. I aspire to inspire. I want to be a living, breathing billboard for what can be done if you decide on and commit to a healthy life change, then put action behind your vision and words.

"To stay motivated, I do something my daddy taught me: I take on a 'warrior mentality,' which means 'commit to victory, no quitting allowed.' This journey has taught me to only compete against myself and never demand perfection from myself, just progress. I advise others to learn to live by the motto 'Meet or beat,' and set your daily goals based on your accomplishments of the previous day. Always remember that you are NOT on a diet, but that you are living an intentional, happier, and healthier lifestyle, full of purpose.

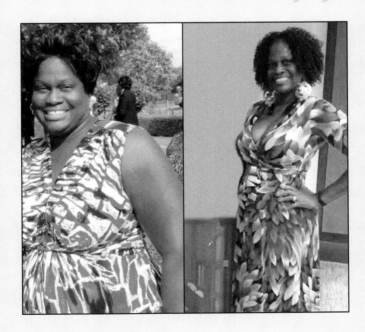

Miche lost 70 pounds and says, "I have learned to not only live but to love myself in the process!"

My journey with green smoothies has been truly phenomenal. It may sound like a cliché, but it has saved and transformed my life. I had lost two loved ones, was overweight and unhappy with the way I looked, had allergies and a cough that lasted about seven months before I started drinking green smoothies. On top of which, I couldn't sleep and had a lump in my breast. I had tried everything there is, including exercise and Zumba, but by not eating right and not knowing the right supplements to use for my body, there were no improvements.

"I started on this journey weighing 230 pounds, and now, two years later, I am 70 pounds lighter at 160. My lump is gone, my allergies are nonexistent (only when I skip smoothies for more than three days do I experience some stuffiness), I sleep better, and the cough has stopped. I don't even have to use face powder because I have the green smoothie glow.

"I am proud of myself. I can take pictures without hiding parts of my body, and my energy is totally awesome. Everyone I interact with is always complimenting me, and they want to know what I did. The support is tremendous on the JJ's Facebook page.

"I joined the VIP Group (see Appendix B), where JJ acts as our personal nutritionist. The highlights include hearing directly from JJ two or three times a month and being able to ask her and her team questions every day. It was the best investment I made for myself. Every day, we get free information about the types of foods to eat, cookbooks, supplements that are right for our bodies, and monthly challenges to help us stay on top of our game. We simply have no excuse not to do it and get it right.

"JJ truly cares about us, and I am so happy I had the privilege of meeting her and her team. This has been nothing short of amazing for me. I have made new friends and have connected with many people who are on a similar journey. The camaraderie provides an awesome family feeling—there is so much love that you can actually feel it coming through cyberspace.

"In May 2015, I was faced with another major setback in my life. I was in the middle of a separation after twenty-two years of marriage, and if it wasn't for the support and being able to come to the Facebook page and get my everyday inspiration and encouragement from so many of my friends in the group and countless others, I don't know what I would have done. I am still standing. I thank God for their support as well that from my inner circle and my two beautiful daughters who have stood with me and supported me continually. I have to do it for them as well.

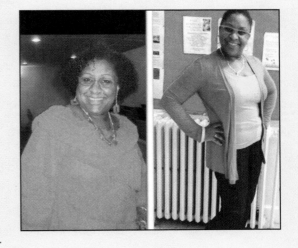

"I have learned that no matter what comes your way to never give up, to stand strong, and always, always think about yourself and what is best for you, because at the end of the day if you don't take care of you, you may as well just curl up and die. I have learned to *live,* and not only live but to love myself in the process.

"A lot of people don't know how important it is to detox your body from all the toxins in food and the environment and also from the negative people in your life, so I have made it my mission to educate and pay it forward to all with whom I come in contact. I share the good news about green smoothies to all those who need it because it is truly a lifesaver to thousands. I am happy and privileged to say that I drink green smoothies for life."

Marla lost 110 pounds and got her motivation back!

" Have you ever had a time in your life when you couldn't see a reason to get up and out? I have. It wasn't because of illness or depression, it was mainly because I didn't have the motivation. Yes, I'm a mother, wife, business owner, housekeeper, nurse . . . the list goes on and on. There have been piles and piles of stress dropped on me, some of which I have placed on myself needlessly. With this stress came poor time management. As the time was tied up, so was the meal preparation. I had gotten to a point where if ramen noodles and butter worked, that's what the family got. Salad? What? That takes too long. Well, forget fruits because they go bad too quickly. We needed something that would stay in the fridge for weeks on end and not go bad . . . hot dogs, bologna, Velveeta, Hawaiian bread chips—oh, and don't forget the soda!

"This had gone on for decades, and heaviness came upon me. Sure, I tried different diet and exercise plans to lose weight, and I would be successful for a while. Then yet another stress would jump on my back, and I would put off the plan . . . for just a little while. I was not able to walk for a long time or distance because my feet and back hurt. I hadn't slept a full night in sixteen years. Sleeping had become more difficult recently because I would wake up at all hours to the numbness and burning in my hands.

"Fast-forward: I am tired, menopause is setting in, and I try to work out but am so lethargic. I see doctors who tell me just to lift weights. Really? I started working out in November and things were okay. I would get on the stationary bike for one to two hours (oh, did I say I was supplementing with caffeine to stay up?) and lift weights. I cut way down on eating . . . I know, I know, just to see the scale go down. In eight weeks' time, I had only lost 8 pounds. Sadness.

"Then, my friend had a post about this Green Cleanse. 'Hmm,' I thought, 'This looks interesting and I need this.' I jumped in. Since that first smoothie—and I do mean first—I have felt energized. I have slept nearly the whole night away. The numbing, burning sensation in my hands is nearly gone, and I even park great distances away to walk to buildings—let the other folks have the 'good' spots.

"I have done JJ's 30-Day Program and to date, I have lost a total of 110 pounds. My hair, skin, and nails are in the best shape they have been in years. I have dropped from a size 22/24 to a size 4/6. Who has ever heard of having energy to spare? Well, that's me! Marla had gone missing in action for over twenty years, but no longer. I smile and laugh freely now. There is still a ways to go on this journey, but I will get there. I feel so blessed to have been given this precious gift. Green smoothies are a mega life-changer. My only hope is that anyone who is searching gets introduced to this healthy lifestyle. **"**

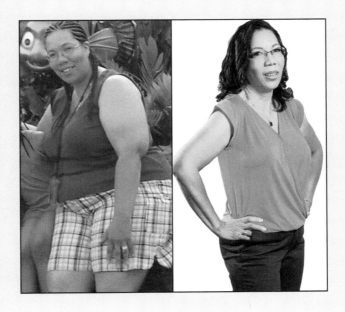

Tameka lost 120 pounds and got her life back!

" I started this amazing journey in April after watching from the sidelines for about two weeks. During those two weeks I made up my mind that I was going to start with the Green Smoothie Cleanse. I said it was the change I was looking for and informed my family of the new lifestyle I was about to embrace! I'm a thirty-year-old woman with polycystic ovarian syndrome (PCOS), a hormonal imbalance that causes weight gain despite dieting and exercise. I was 300 pounds but was blessed not to have any other major health issues. Congestive heart failure, high blood pressure, and diabetes have completely taken a toll on my family, and that's all I could see happening to me as well.

"Day 4 into the full green smoothie cleanse, I started my cycle for the first time on my own in over ten years! PCOS had caused me to have irregular cycles. I would normally go a year or so without my cycle. Medications that the doctors prescribed didn't even work. I had almost given up hope for a second child since I wasn't able to ovulate due to my irregular cycles.

"After completing JJ's 30-Day Program, and drinking green smoothies for four months, my body had regulated itself. I've had a cycle every month since I started! Fast-forward to a year later, I am down 120 pounds and my relationship with food has completely changed! Carbs were my main addiction! I would have dinner with two carbs and no vegetables. But I haven't touched a carb. I look at all food labels and refuse to eat any of the processed foods I used to eat. I haven't had any red meat, sweets, refined foods, saturated foods, white sugar, table salt, or any type of artificial sweetener since I started this amazing journey! JJ Smith and green smoothies have completely changed and saved my life forever!

"I sit back and think of all the years I was upset, depressed, and self-conscious. I was in so much pain from the loose ligaments in both knees. I wouldn't have any energy during the day. I suffered badly from insomnia. I even resented my mom for talking me out of the gastric bypass surgery that I was approved for. Hardest of all, I was unable to have any more children because doctors couldn't balance my hormones. Now I have a chance at having another child. My insomnia medication has been discontinued. My knees haven't had me down due to being in so much pain or giving out on me. My energy is amazing—I haven't needed the daily nap I had become so used to. I'm now grateful to my mother for talking me out of the bypass surgery. I'm on a natural high, and life is so amazing. "

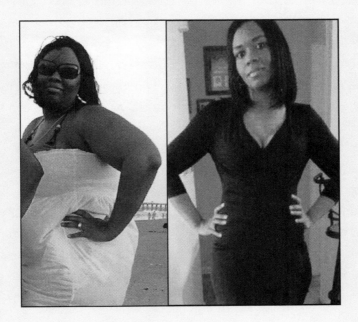

Rashawnda lost 46 pounds and became a healthy BMI and weight and now she can donate a kidney to her dad!

"A brief background on my health: I had an unexplained weight gain of 60 pounds in less than six months about ten years ago. After several tests were done, it was discovered that I had PCOS [polycystic ovary syndrome]. With the weight gain, I then developed high blood pressure and sleep apnea. Having PCOS, along with a history of diabetes on both sides of the family, tripled my odds of developing diabetes. Ever since being diagnosed with PCOS, I was told it would be difficult to lose weight. It was somewhat drilled into my head. And I began to use that as my crutch. I was on every diet and medication possible to lose weight but was never successful in the long term. I think reality began to hit home when my father's kidney function began to dwindle and ultimately failed. And he had to rely on dialysis three times a week.

"I started the Green Smoothie Cleanse journey on January 27 at 184 pounds after my friend recommended it. I was a little apprehensive since I was such a picky eater and never too fond of eating greens. After completing my first cleanse, I lost 13 pounds and gained so much energy. I was definitely a believer! I've been drinking green smoothies for 7¼ months, and so far I've lost close to 46 pounds and am currently a size 4. I am eating clean meals daily and walk at least 3 miles a day. Also, I am no longer on blood pressure medicine and no longer need the CPAP for my sleep apnea.

"The biggest reward of this new lifestyle is that I am now at a healthy BMI and weight so I can donate a kidney to my dad. I was told that my labs show that we are a match, and next week I will go through extensive testing to see if I'll be fit physically for the transplant. JJ and the Facebook group members have been in my corner since Day One, and I thank her so very much for providing me with the tools to take back my health and life.

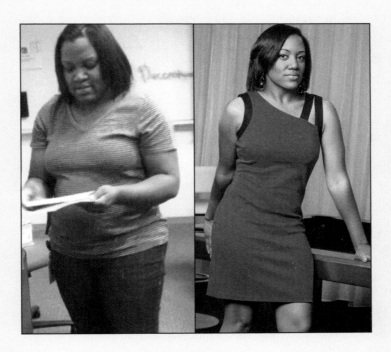

Doris went from a size 14 to a size 6 and lost 40 pounds!

"Just like many others, I have struggled with my weight all my life. There was not a time I can remember that I was not on a diet. About twenty years ago, I started to have issues with my back, and after many procedures, physical therapy, and surgeries, I had a spinal fusion. Unfortunately, I had complications and I became unable to work anymore. The weight started to creep up on me, and I did my best to keep it under control, but it was difficult now that I was unable to do the many physical things I used to be able to do.

"Fast-forward to August. I was on my way to a wake for the father of a childhood friend, when I was rear-ended on the highway by a texting driver. The force of the impact sent my upper back into spasm and ruptured four discs in my neck. In constant pain and now depressed, my weight ballooned to an all-time high. In January, my doctor diagnosed me with prediabetes. I was frightened, and although she gave me a detailed diet plan to help me lose the weight I so desperately needed, I could not stick with it. The cravings I had for sugar, salt, and carbs were overwhelming, and I failed miserably at every turn to lose the weight.

"Then, one day in March, a dear friend who had been there for me and helped me when my faith was wavering, posted that she and her husband were about to do a Green Smoothie Cleanse. Intrigued, I contacted her about it, bought the book that same day, shopped that night, and started my first cleanse the very next morning. I felt that God had given me this path to follow, and I was going to give it my all!

"Using the tools JJ Smith gave me, I embarked on a journey of renewed health, weight loss, and happiness I had not experienced in years. With every passing day, I felt better, my depression lifted, my skin cleared up, and I slept better. The next time I had my blood work done, my doctor informed me that my prediabetes was nonexistent. I went from a tight size 14 to a size 6 pants, and lost 40 pounds. In five short months, I got my health and my foxy back.

I will always have chronic pain, back issues, and limitations on what I can do physically, but I am no longer a slave to my sugar, salt, and carb cravings. I now have the tools to give my body what it needs, so I can be the healthiest version of me possible. "

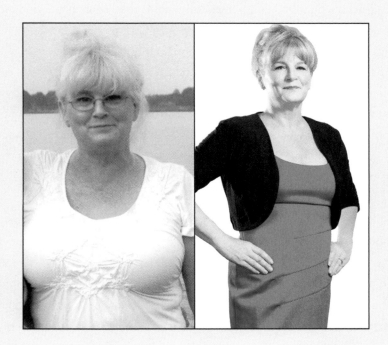

Melodee lost 50 pounds!

"For years, I had struggled with my weight and recurrent urinary tract infections, but otherwise I considered myself fairly healthy. During my second pregnancy, I suffered with sciatica. After I delivered the baby, the everyday excruciating pain subsided, but my back began to hurt with a dull ache that worsened if I stood for long periods of time or if I did a lot of bending. My doctor said it was still sciatica, but I refused to take pain killers because I just don't like being dependent on medicine. I didn't have blood pressure, heart, or cholesterol problems, or diabetes. I had tried a lot of stuff to lose weight—pills, shakes, fad diets, you name it, I've tried it. Sometimes, I was successful and would lose a few pounds, only to gain them back once I quit. I can't say that my weight has ever been linked to my self-esteem, because I'm pretty confident in who I am no matter what size I am. However, I was an emotional eater. Stress to me equaled food! And let's just say, I am stressed a lot. Much of it is my own fault. I am a giver, so it is hard for me to tell people no, even when it's at the expense of me resting or taking care of my own responsibilities.

"On Friday, February 28, I made up my mind that I was going to start my green smoothie journey on Monday, March 3. I took my before pictures and when I did, OMGreen! My stomach looked like I was six months pregnant! I was upset with myself for looking like that! About six days into the green smoothie life, I noticed that my back pain had lessened quite tremendously and I had energy like I've never had before. On Day 8, I posted a pic of me on February 28 and a pic of me on March 10. The results that I experienced were phenomenal. On that very day, more than fifty people contacted me about how the changes in my looks inspired them to get the book and start the cleanse.

"But the biggest change for me during my green smoothie journey was what happened on the inside. I found out who I really am! I'm black, beautiful, intelligent, and real, and I have a right to live my best, healthy life. As of today, at least two hundred people that I know have seen my results and the changes in my skin and my overall being, and have decided that they want to be about this life, too. I have completed the 30-Day Program to learn how to incorporate green smoothies into my daily lifestyle and I am currently down 50 pounds. My white blood cell count is normal for the first time in years. I feel good, I look good, and I am good! Green smoothies have changed my whole life!"

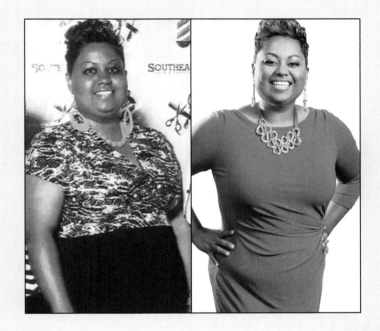

Deborah lost 65 pounds!

"For years I hid from cameras and draped my body in big dresses, tops, long skirts or pants. At 5'1" and 198 pounds, size 18, I was all butt, gut and boobs with skinny legs. So when I wore anything that showed my legs I looked out of balance. Since February, by following the green smoothie program of replacing two meals a day with smoothies and eating a healthy dinner, I have a new love for the benefits of this healthy lifestyle and life in general. But the real success story is that green smoothies have helped me lay the foundation for breaking the bad health cycle which has already claimed several of my

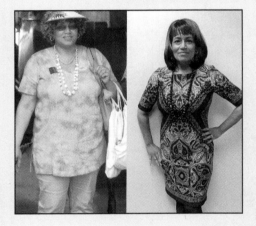

family members: diabetes, high cholesterol, high blood pressure, strokes—just to name a few.

"At sixty-four years old, I am now the matriarch of my family, and I want to be available for them—to help my remaining family members become healthy. The weight and inches lost is an outcome of healthy living after years of trying so many diets to only regain the weight I dropped and then some.

"Now with green smoothies, I am enjoying the benefits of improving my health, mental wellness, and getting my sexy back. My cholesterol level has dropped from 212 to 132. I no longer need my asthma and inflammation reduction medicine. My medical digestive issues have disappeared. I have energy where I was constantly out of breath and exhausted.

"There are visual differences: I have dropped 65 pounds and have learned how to maintain that weight loss! I now wear size 4 tops, 2 bottoms and X-smalls in clothing. Mental difference, I face life with more confidence and with peace by having clear-headed thinking. I know this is a lifelong journey where I cannot stray from JJ's guidance, without seeing negative aspects creep back in my life. Evidence is in the pictures. Thank you, JJ, for sharing your advice on how to detox the body and eat healthy! I love all my Green Smoothie Cleanse family."

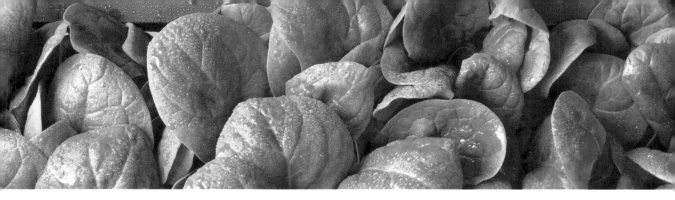

PART 4
AN OVERVIEW OF THE DHEMM SYSTEM: A PERMANENT WEIGHT-LOSS SYSTEM

After you complete the 30-Day Program, you should transition to the DHEMM System, a permanent weight-loss philosophy that will help you reach your desired weight. The 30-Day Program meal plans are very prescriptive and take the guesswork out of eating, snacking, and incorporating green smoothies into your regimen. The DHEMM System, on the other hand, takes a more comprehensive approach to weight loss and addresses more complex issues, including balancing hormones and the psychology of weight loss. So most people begin by jump-starting their weight loss with the 10-Day Green Smoothie Cleanse. After the 10 days, you follow the 30-Day Program to learn how to incorporate green smoothies into your regimen for life so you can continue to lose weight. As you look to reach your ideal weight, the DHEMM System provides all the advanced approaches to weight loss that are commonly overlooked by traditional dieting. The DHEMM System addresses topics like detoxing, balancing your hormones, and moving (exercising). This should allow you to lose the weight you desire to and keep it off.

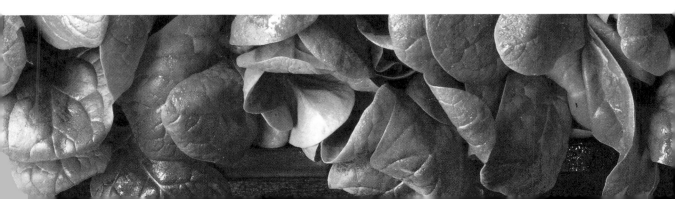

THE DHEMM SYSTEM STANDS FOR:

- *DETOX:* Use one of the many detox methods described in this book

- *HORMONAL BALANCE:* Optimize your hormones for weight loss

- *EAT CLEAN:* Eat healthy, whole, and unprocessed foods

- *MENTAL MASTERY:* Achieve the right mind-set to stay motivated

- *MOVE:* Get moving and increase your physical activity

The DHEMM System makes weight loss more effortless, melting excess fat from your body, especially from stubborn areas like the hips, thighs, and belly. Through detoxing the body and enjoying clean, healthy meals, you can lose the weight you desire. Even if obesity runs in your family, you can break that hereditary cycle with this new approach to managing your weight. You can't change your genes, but by simply eating smart, you can manage how your body functions to optimize your health.

The DHEMM System is a complete weight-management program designed to help your body clear out old toxic waste that contributes to excess fat in the body. By following the DHEMM System, you can learn what many people don't know and what celebrities pay thousands of dollars to famous doctors to learn. You will learn how to detox and eat in a manner that helps your body lose weight and achieve optimum health.

The DHEMM System teaches you to eat clean by enjoying tasty, satisfying foods, including green smoothies. I believe food is to be enjoyed and should help us not only maintain great health but also help us stay slim and lean. Following the DHEMM System, you will give your body the quality nutrition it needs while cleansing your cells on an ongoing basis. Vitamins, minerals, and other nutrients will be absorbed by your body more efficiently, allowing your cells to become like new as you begin to look and feel younger. Your skin will begin to look more youthful because your cells become tighter and healthier. You will get healthy from the inside out.

DETOX

With the DHEMM System, you learn various detox methods to ensure that you release toxins on a regular basis because releasing toxins releases weight. Some readers have already detoxed using the 10-Day Green Smoothie Cleanse or the other methods listed in Part 2 of this book. Remember, detoxing is something you must do consistently.

WHY WE DETOX

Many people go from one diet to another because the results, no matter what the diet emphasizes—high protein vs. no carbs, for example—are often temporary. But as I've written in the detox section of this book, most traditional diets overlook an important factor for losing weight permanently: You must get rid of excess toxins in the body. Without purging your body of its toxins, it's difficult for the body to shed pounds. The more toxins you take in or get exposed to every day, the more toxins you store as fat cells in the body. Toxins stored in fat cells are difficult to get rid of through dieting alone. As I explained in Part I, you must first detoxify the body. When the body is overloaded with toxins, the body transfers its energy away from burning calories and uses that energy to detoxify the body. However, when the body is efficiently detoxifying and getting rid of toxins, the energy can be used to burn fat, which is what we want.

The only way to get rid of toxins stored in fat cells is to detoxify the body. Cutting calories does not detox the body. So you must focus on detoxing the body if you want to permanently lose weight. Once you rid the body of toxins, you can best metabolize the food you eat without leaving behind excess waste that results in weight gain.

WHAT ARE TOXINS?

I often get asked, "What exactly are toxins?" and I typically respond by saying toxins make us fat and they make us sick! They are the missing piece to the puzzle as to why we can't lose weight and why we feel so unhealthy and tired!

A toxin is any substance that irritates or creates harmful effects in the body or mind. Toxins are everywhere, and we are unknowingly filling our bodies with them every day. There are two types of toxins: environmental toxins and internal toxins.

- Environmental toxins are found outside the body/mind and include pollutants, smog, prescription medications, hormones/birth control pills, household cleaners, food additives, pesticides.

- Internal toxins are found inside the body/mind and include bacterial/yeast/fungal overgrowth, parasite infections, chronic worry or fear, food allergies, and dental or medical implants such as implants from cosmetic surgeries, joint replacements, or mercury dental fillings.

Toxins are really hard to avoid, but you can help your body get rid of some of them. Every person on the planet contains residues of toxic chemicals or metals in their tissues. Over 80,000 new chemicals have been introduced since the turn of the twentieth century, and most have never been tested for safety or for how they interact in the human body. Our air is toxic; our water is polluted; our food is depleted of nutrients and packed with poisonous chemicals and hormones. Not only that, but our minds and hearts often get polluted also, which is why detoxing helps us in our mind, body, and spirit.

Toxins create a heavy burden in the body, which causes many of the body's systems to malfunction. The buildup of toxins overwhelms the body's vital organs and other systems, creating an array of health problems including fatigue, memory loss, premature aging, skin eruptions/acne, depression, arthritis, hormone imbalances, chronic fatigue, anxiety, emotional disorders, muscle and joint pain, cancers, heart disease, and much, much more.

As I gained weight in my thirties, I learned that although my metabolism was beginning to slow due to aging, that wasn't the real reason why I couldn't lose weight. I learned that my excess weight was not all fat; some of it was waste in my body— excess toxic waste caused by years of poor eating, which lead to inflammation, fluid retention, and intestinal waste in my colon.

It's important to understand that we're all toxic, which is one of the biggest reasons so many people are overweight. Just because you are overweight does not guarantee that you have toxic overload, and just because you are thin does not mean that you do not have a toxic overload. We have to evaluate our toxic overload individually regardless of whether we are slim or fat. However, it is rare that an overweight person who rids the body of excess toxins does not lose weight. Please know that getting rid of the fat by exercising or dieting doesn't necessarily get rid of the toxins. Toxins just get reabsorbed by your body, creating new fat cells that hinder your ability to lose weight permanently.

Signs of toxic overload in the body include the following:

- Bloating and gas
- Constipation
- Indigestion
- Low energy/fatigue
- Brain fog/depression

- Weight gain
- Chronic pain
- Infections
- Allergies
- Headaches

One of the most commonly held myths today is that the body can detoxify itself and does not need any help. You may have heard that the body can eliminate toxins on its own. Our body does naturally try to eliminate toxins, but overexposure to any of them will slow down the body's detoxification systems. The reality is that you can assist the body in detoxifying and eliminating toxins that causes weight gain and harm your health. You can and should detoxify and cleanse the body if you want to live better and live longer. Yes, toxins are real, they do exist, and the good news is that there are many ways to eliminate them from the body.

I believe the most effective weight-loss programs should focus on both fat loss and detoxification. Detoxification is a total-body cleansing process that removes toxins from the body. Detoxification is critical to losing fat because many of the toxins the body holds on to are stored in fat cells. When you detoxify the body, toxins stored in fat cells are released and eliminated from the body so they don't cause weight gain and illness. Therefore, weight loss that includes detoxification results in not only fat loss but also overall improved health and wellness. In this book I share twenty-one ways to detoxify the body including colonics, saunas, body brushing, and many others so that you can reduce the toxic overload in your body, which hinders your ability to lose weight permanently.

HORMONAL IMBALANCE

With the DHEMM System, both men and women will learn to balance your hormones for weight loss. The DHEMM System teaches you to:

- Discover the five hormones that slow weight loss, and take a self-assessment quiz to determine if you have them
- Learn how to get tested for hormonal imbalances and learn which specific blood or saliva tests to request from your doctor
- Find out the best natural supplements and treatments to optimize your hormones for weight loss
- Learn how to work with your doctor to treat and correct hormonal imbalances and watch the pounds melt away

The mantra of "eat less and exercise more" is ineffective for many people who want to lose weight. We know that the no-carb, low carb, no-fat, low-fat crazes of the eighties and nineties were hit-or-miss in terms of results. Fortunately, we now have better scientific information on more important factors that help us lose weight: hormonal balance.

Welcome to the world of understanding your hormones, the little messengers that control your appetite, metabolism, and how much weight you gain or lose. Please note that if you are a woman over the age of thirty-five, there are three key sex hormones (estrogen, progesterone, and testosterone) that play a role in weight gain.

It is essential to understand how hormones play a role in maintaining our weight. To explain it, I will paraphrase some of the detailed information I give in *Lose Weight Without Dieting or Working Out*. Hormones control almost every aspect of how we gain and lose weight. Some hormones tell you you're hungry, some tell you you're full; some tell your body what to do with the food that is eaten, whether to use it as fuel for energy or store it as fat, which causes us to gain weight. Hormones are responsible for metabolizing fat. By controlling your hormones, you can control your weight.

Hormones impact how you feel, how you look, and most important, how you maintain your weight and health. When your hormones are balanced properly, you will have great health, beauty, and vibrancy. When your hormones are imbalanced, you have mood swings, you crave unhealthy foods, and you feel sluggish and lethargic.

As I've shared before, I once had an unexplained weight gain of 30 pounds, practically overnight, in just a few months. If I ate a Big Mac, I gained a pound by the next day. But today I can easily eat 2,000 calories of nutrient-rich foods a day, without exercising, and still maintain my current weight. None of this would be possible without finely tuned hormones that accelerate my metabolism and cause me to burn fat as opposed to storing fat. I'm happy to reap the benefits of a stronger metabolism now, but for years my hormones were working against me. I didn't understand much about them years ago, but now I know how to ensure that they work in my favor.

HORMONES CONTROL YOUR APPETITE

There are certain hormones that balance hunger and fullness in the brain that are key to permanent weight control. If you were never hungry, losing weight would be very easy. If you properly control the hormones that are directly affected by what you eat, you will not be hungry between meals and will have sufficient fuel and energy for the day. This will expedite fat loss.

Feeling hungry is one of the most powerful urges we have. When you feel hungry, everything else is secondary to getting food into your system. This is because the brain becomes desperate to get the energy it needs to function.

There are hormones that control your weight, often called metabolic hormones, brain messenger chemicals called neuropeptides, and messenger molecules of the immune system called cytokines, produced in the fat cells, white blood cells, and liver cells. All of these components work together to communicate to the organs and tissues responsible for managing your weight and keeping you alive. Good communication results in a healthy metabolism. These finely tuned systems determine your health and metabolism. They are what tell you that you are full and to stop eating, making the difference between whether you gain or lose weight.

Let's see how these complex messenger signals work. When your stomach is empty, one of the chemical messengers secretes hormones that tell your body and brain you are hungry. Your brain then prepares the stomach to receive some food. When you eat, the food enters the gut and releases yet more hormones, preparing it for digestion. As the food makes its way into your bloodstream, more messages coordinate your metabolism, telling your pancreas to produce insulin. Your fat cells then send hormonal messages back to your brain to stop eating, along with signals from your stomach that you are full. Your liver then metabolizes or processes fat and sugar and helps use it for energy or store the excess as fat.

Your body can't work the way it's supposed to if any one of the hormones is out of sync. You have to be able to naturally optimize how all your hormones work as opposed to trying to address one at a time. They are too closely integrated to address one; if one is out of sync, then there are already other chemical imbalances in the body.

5 HORMONAL IMBALANCES THAT SLOW WEIGHT LOSS

- Insulin resistance
- Polycystic Ovary Syndrome (PCOS)
- Hypothyroid
- High cortisol
- Estrogen dominance

When you learn the DHEMM System (and once you have your hormones tested you will be able to identify the 5 hormonal imbalances, and learn how to get treated for them. Once you balance your hormones, you will find that weight loss will be easier and more effortless.

Chronic hormonal imbalances cause you to gain weight and feel moody and fatigued. You will need to detoxify and cleanse your body—and your kitchen and household—of the toxic waste that causes you to get fat. You will need to provide your body with healing foods that allow your metabolism to work as a fat-burning machine instead of a fat-storing machine. When your hormones are functioning at their optimal levels, your body is at peak performance and maintains your healthy, ideal weight.

To determine if you are hormonally imbalanced, you should consult a trained health-care provider who can, through a series of laboratory tests (sometimes called a hormonal panel), understand your current hormone levels. The two most common types are saliva testing and blood testing.

For a more detailed discussion of how hormones affect weight, see *Lose Weight Without Dieting or Working Out*.

EAT CLEAN

Let's talk about EATING. On the DHEMM System, you will not only eat well but you will continue to retrain your body to desire healthy, natural foods. With the DHEMM System, you will never count calories or have to follow expensive, bland meal plans.

When you eat foods that are primarily natural, whole, raw, or organic, your body can more effectively digest and metabolize these foods. Healthy foods are recognizable by the body and can be broken down, whereas unnatural foods and ingredients cannot be broken down and will actually cause weight gain, bloating, and other ailments. The healthiest foods are those that are the easiest for the body to digest—they are effectively broken down and utilized and leave little waste or toxins in the body.

The goal of the DHEMM System is to eat "clean and balanced." "Clean" foods are primarily natural, whole, raw, or organic—foods that the body can effectively digest and utilize for energy without leaving excess waste or toxins in the body. "Clean" foods include lean proteins, good carbs, and healthy fats. "Balanced" foods mean that you eat protein every time you eat a carbohydrate. So, if you have carbohydrates, you want to always include protein. It is a very simple but effective method for preventing insulin spikes and aiding the body in burning fat.

You have probably heard a lot about the need to eat "whole foods." What are whole foods? Whole foods are foods that are fresh and unprocessed and remain almost exactly in the form that they were found in nature. Whole foods include beans, vegetables, whole grains, fruits, nuts, and seeds. As we stated earlier, the quicker your body is able to break down and digest food, the less waste matter it leaves behind that eventually turns into fat cells in the body. Additionally, the longer it takes the body to break food down to digest it, the longer you'll feel full and satisfied throughout the day.

You also hear a lot about organic foods, which are free from chemical preservatives, additives, hormones, pesticides, and antibiotics. Fresh organic foods are far less toxic than highly processed and packaged/frozen foods. Organic foods support good health and help you maintain your ideal weight as well as detoxify the body. Fresh organic fruits, vegetables, whole grains, and meats are best for you. Frozen fruits and vegetables retain many vitamins and often don't contain as many preservatives as packaged and canned foods, but they lack vital enzymes needed for the body to digest them properly. Frozen dinners and canned, boxed, and instant foods are the least healthy options because they often contain sugar, salt, preservatives, and unhealthy fats.

THE THREE FOUNDATION FOODS FOR HEALTHY EATING

I've often heard that 80 percent of weight loss is what you eat. The three foundation foods for the DHEMM System are lean proteins, good carbohydrates (carbs), and healthy fats. What you eat is the most important factor in losing weight. You can do all the exercising you want, but if you do not feed your body the necessary foods with the right nutrients that your body requires, then you will hinder your progress toward your weight-loss goals. Knowing what to eat is foundational to staying slim. Eating a healthy, well-balanced meal with lean proteins, good carbohydrates, and healthy fats will help you lose weight and keep it off.

Over the years, I've learned that most people don't know the differences between proteins, carbohydrates, and fats. For instance, many people don't know that fruits and vegetables are carbohydrates. It's important for you to start to think of all foods as either proteins, carbs, or fats. This information is critical to managing your weight long term because each type of food has different hormonal impacts affecting weight gain.

- Lean proteins. One of the most effective nutrients for speeding up metabolism and building muscle in the body is protein. Protein boosts the caloric burn while it is being digested and helps to build muscle that also helps burn calories. Examples of lean proteins include eggs, fish, lean poultry, or lean beef (preferably organic and grass- or range-fed meat).

- Good carbs. Good Carbohydrates, particularly those found in their natural form, contain most of the essential nutrients that keep you healthy, give you energy, and turn up your metabolism. Examples include fruits, vegetables, whole grains, beans, nuts, and seeds. Bad carbs are considered white potatoes, breads, pastas, etc.

- Healthy fats. Healthy fats, also known as unsaturated fats, are the good fats—those that have omega-3 fatty acids that help speed up your metabolism and help your body burn fat more quickly. Examples include fish oil; extra-virgin olive oil; cold-pressed plant oils, such as grapeseed oil and sesame oil; nuts and seeds; and coconut.

With the DHEMM System, you will learn hundreds of foods that are primarily natural, whole, raw, or organic. They are high in fiber and omega-3 fatty acids and great for weight loss and optimum health.

MENTAL MASTERY

With the DHEMM System, you'll learn the mental strategies for weight-loss success. Weight loss is a process. Mental mastery helps you understand the psychological stages required to not only lose weight but to maintain your weight loss also.

Weight loss happens in the mind before it happens in the body. You really can think yourself thin. No matter how much you learn about nutrition, if you don't have the right mind-set, the right mental focus, you won't achieve your results.

After helping folks lose over 2 million pounds in two years, I've watched individuals start at the same time and some mentally lock in and achieve their weight-loss goals, while others still lose and gain the same 20 pounds over and over again. However, some have discovered the mental strategies, the focus, the discipline to succeed at weight loss.

Mental mastery will help folks understand if they are *interested* in losing weight or truly *committed* to losing weight? How do you know if you are interested or committed? If you're truly committed, you'll do whatever it takes and make the necessary sacrifices to lose weight. That's being uncomfortable from time to time. Maybe that means you have to go to lunch by yourself sometimes? You have to invest in learning how to help your unique body lose weight. You truly have to commit to weight loss until you achieve your goal. People fail not because of lack of interest or desire but lack of commitment.

MENTAL MASTERY TIPS

In order to ensure success on your weight-loss journey, here are a few tips to help you stay mentally focused and motivated:

Make your health a priority. First, decide that your health is one of the top priorities in your life. If you prepare your mind and absorb the knowledge offered to you in this book, you will have all the power you need to become your best self and transform your life in every way. Whether you're running a household, a company, or both, know that today begins the journey toward your most amazing, beautiful self. It is time to treat your body as the greatest gift that you have. It is time to shine as the person you were always meant to be. When you have a healthy and positive energy in life, amazing things like love, joy, success, and wealth come your way. Every interaction at work, church, home, or in the streets can be simply magnetic. Get healthy, lose weight, and watch your entire life begin to change for the better.

List the reasons why you want to lose weight. Be sure the list includes both scale and non-scale victories like more energy, better sleep, less cravings. Give serious thought to this list and ensure that each reason reflects your true goals and desires and that the list is meaningful to you. The reasons should be highly personal and not meant to please anyone but yourself. These become your personal motivators. Read them every day. You may even want to post them at work or carry them in your purse or wallet on an index card. You will need to remind yourself of these motivators to keep yourself focused.

Visualize your healthy, thin body. Can you envision what you will look like when you're thinner and healthier? Visualize your perfect body and get comfortable with the idea it will be yours by the end of this program. Everything in life is made up of energy, including your thoughts. Positive thoughts attract positive energy. Negative thoughts attract negative energy. What you think is what you become. If you think of yourself as slim and healthy, you will begin to move in the direction of being thin and healthy. Don't think about being overweight, think about being thin. See yourself as having an attractive, sexy, energetic body. Allow your thoughts to work with your efforts of changing your eating habits so that you accelerate your progress, having everything in your life working with you, not against you.

Engage in positive self-talk. Thoughts and feelings turn into actions, and actions into reality. Remember, you are beginning a new chapter in your life. Let me encourage you right now to get started with your journey. Many ask, "How do I start?" or "How do I get there?" Well, it begins with positive self-talk. You want to stop thinking and saying negative things about yourself. You are not fat, lazy, ugly, or sick. Your true self is naturally thin, beautiful, and healthy. If you have negative thoughts about yourself, you'll attract negative people and outcomes in your life. If you say that you can never lose weight, you're exactly right: you won't. If you say you can, your subconscious mind believes that and begins to move your actions in the direction of losing weight.

Don't obsess over the scale. Don't let your bathroom scale ruin your motivation. Weighing yourself frequently can be confusing because your weight will fluctuate, so focus on how your clothes look and feel on your body. Scales are reliable over the long haul but give you inaccurate day-to-day reads. Weight fluctuations can be caused by hormonal changes or fluid shifts and can lead to unnecessary disappointment. It can show gains or losses that are not there because most basic scales can't tell the difference between fat, muscle, and water weight. Your weight also fluctuates by several pounds throughout the day, and weighing yourself too much will only be confusing and discouraging. Plan on weighing yourself only once a week at the same time of day and wearing the same clothing or no clothing (naked is best). Focus on losing inches and on how you begin to feel, not just on pounds. With this program, you will be doing great things for your body and health. The number on the scale will take care of itself. Be happy with losing 1 to 2 pounds per week. If you do this for two months, you will be down by 16 pounds.

Focus on losing body fat, not just weight. Losing pounds is nice, but what's key to getting in a smaller dress or pants size is losing body fat. It's fine to have a weight goal to use as a guideline, but also focus on measuring and monitoring overall body fat as a percentage of overall weight. This will ensure that you lose fat, not muscle. Healthful body-fat percentages for men begin at about 8 percent, 22 percent for women. These percentages will keep you in a healthy, safe zone that will lower your risk for disease. If you only have a regular scale and want to get detailed body-fat measurements, you can invest in a home body-fat scale. A decent one will cost you $100 to $200. I own one by Tanita that measures weight, body-fat percentages, and muscle mass, and helps me get the best picture of my overall health. Once you begin to measure your body fat, you will be able to track the loss of the thing you really want to lose.

Take a picture! Looking at before and after pictures of your new face and body can be highly motivating. Of course, you'll be getting comments and compliments from friends, family, and coworkers, but nothing is as special as seeing with your very own eyes your new healthy, beautiful body. Health is important, but I understand your need to improve your physical appearance as well. So get out the camera and take photos as you progress along your weight-loss journey.

The reason some people look and feel better than others is that they work at it. Why do you think celebrities look so fabulous despite their age? It's because they are constantly thinking about their appearance. Their livelihood depends upon how good they look. However, anyone can commit to looking fabulous all the time. You can make the choice to eat whole, healthy foods instead of junk foods, stay active, drink lots of water, and get plenty of rest and relaxation. Yes, it takes more work and discipline to look great as you age, but you will reap the benefits of being your best, beautiful self.

MOVE

It's time to get moving even if we can't get to a gym. Most of us spend the majority of the day sitting in our cars, watching TV, or sitting in front of a computer. Our bodies suffer because we sit for fourteen or fifteen hours or more every day. It weakens our heart, slows our metabolism, and weakens our muscle strength. We used to sit when we needed a break from our hectic day, but now we sit over 80 percent of our waking hours.

The way we diet and exercise today is ineffective. We can't just be sedentary for fifteen hours a day and think thirty minutes on the treadmill, only burning about 250 calories, is sufficient physical activity. We should be burning calories through constant physical activity throughout each day. Additionally, when we try to diet by selectively eliminating entire food groups, we often fail because we need all the foundation foods if our bodies are to stay healthy and lean. Our bodies thrive off nourishment and sustenance, not starvation and deprivation. A decade ago, there weren't half as many gyms as there are currently, and yet we didn't struggle with obesity the way we do today. A decade ago, people moved more. They moved to find food, they moved while they worked, and they moved for recreation. The modern electronic age has made us lazier than ever. At work, we don't even walk right down the hall to talk to a coworker. Instead, we use email or text messages. Our fingers are the only body parts that might possibly be gaining muscle strength and endurance. And that has to change.

I've said it before: the DHEMM System isn't an anti-exercise program nor would I ever suggest that you do not exercise. Exercise is great for your overall cardiovascular health but is not a major factor in weight loss. In this book, we discuss the real factors that produce rapid and sustained weight loss, such as eating clean and balanced. More physical activity throughout each day is key to eliminating excess body fat. In short, when you move consistently throughout the day, your body does a better job of burning calories throughout the day. So, the goal is simple: Get moving and become more active, and you will enhance both your weight-loss efforts and your overall health. And getting moving does not necessarily mean going to the gym.

The DHEMM System provides numerous ways to burn calories throughout the day doing everyday activities, as well as tips for achieving a higher level of fitness. You burn calories while you run after the kids, usher churchgoers to their seats, or shop the aisles of your local grocery store. What we won't focus on is going to the gym or working out as the primary method for getting physically active. If you're like me, you struggle to find time to "go somewhere to work out." Going to the gym to work out for an hour does not necessarily make us physically active. Being physically active involves the big and small movements we make throughout each day.

Do not let going to the gym be the only way you focus on getting moving. The goal is to make small changes in your personal and professional life that are easy to do with minimal planning and commitment. As an example, a client of mine purchased a minicycle, a set of pedals that sits on the floor or under a desk. Her goal was to use it while she sat and watched her favorite television drama. She said she kept the resistance pretty low so it wasn't too strenuous but she constantly pedaled very slowly. As a result, she lost 2 pounds in the first week. So she doubled the amount of time she pedaled on the minicycle while watching television and lost 3 pounds the second week. It became an easy habit because she would get in a rhythm and forget she was still pedaling after a while.

The DHEMM System will provide numerous ways to simply get moving without working out or going to the gym. I want to encourage you to live life the way it was meant to be lived: active, engaged, and as a full participant. Get out of your chair, get on your feet, and go live life. Since the majority of our weight and health problems can be eliminated by following the detox guidelines, clean and balanced food recommendations, and the get-moving tips outlined in the DHEMM System, you can achieve optimal health. You will enjoy your new body, energy, health, and well-being. Get excited about your new life. It is not just about weight loss—it's a journey toward optimal health and wellness. You'll love the way it transforms your body, and you'll be thrilled with your results.

To learn more about the DHEMM System, you can purchase *Lose Weight Without Dieting or Working Out* or join JJ's Private VIP Group at www.JJSmithOnline.com.

CONCLUSION

I want to say congrats on taking back control of your health and your weight so that you can live your best life! You are on your way. This is a journey that will change your life—it's *not* a diet but a lifestyle! I would like to encourage you to make time to nourish your inner spirit and soul by giving your body the rest and relaxation it needs to stay strong and healthy. You have given yourself a wonderful gift of optimal health and wellness.

My own commitment to this lifestyle is unwavering due to the amazing results that I have experienced. My forty-plus-year-old body always feels wonderful—youthful and energetic. I never worry about putting on excess weight or returning to the poor state of health that I had in my twenties and thirties. I do not have some special gene that keeps me slim. I could gain excess weight like the next person without this system of healthy living. This lifestyle has benefited thousands who have had some great successes as well. I know that you can—and will—reach your ideal weight and greatest health!

Remember that you have the power to change your life, and now with the information in this book, you have the tools to turn your dreams into reality. Every day is the beginning of the rest of your life. You are in control of what happens today. Start dreaming about a sexy, beautiful body and watch it become reality. You have power over your body and your life, so live life with passion, because you only get one!

I always close my books with my *10 Commandments for Looking Young and Feeling Great.*

1. *Thou shalt love thyself.* Self-love is essential to survival. There is no successful, authentic relationship with others without self-love. We cannot water the land from a dry well. Self-love is not selfish or self-indulgent. We have to take care of our needs first so we can give to others from abundance.

2. *Thou shalt take responsibility for thine own health and well-being.* If you want to be healthy, have more energy, and feel great, you must take the time to learn what is involved and apply it to your own life. You have to watch what goes into your mouth, how much exercise and physical activity you get, and what thoughts you're thinking throughout the day.

3. *Thou shalt sleep.* Sleep and rest is the body's way of recharging the system. Sleep is the easiest yet most underrated activity for healing the body. Lack of sleep definitely saps your glow and instantly ages you, giving you puffy red eyes with dark circles under them.

4. *Thou shalt detoxify and cleanse the body.* Detoxifying the body means ridding the body of wastes and toxins so that you can speed up weight loss and restore great health. Releasing toxins releases weight.

5. *Thou shalt remember that a healthy body is a sexy body.* Real women's bodies look beautiful! A healthy body is a beautiful body. It's about getting healthy and having style and confidence and wearing clothes that match your body type.

6. *Thou shalt eat healthy, natural, whole foods.* Healthy eating can turn back the hands of time and return the body to a more youthful state. When you eat natural foods, you simply look and feel better. You keep the body clean at the cellular level and look radiant despite your age. Eating healthy should be part of your "beauty regimen."

7. *Thou shalt embrace healthy aging.* The goal is not to stop the aging process but to embrace it. Healthy aging is staying healthy as you age, which is looking and feeling great despite your age.

8. ***Thou shalt commit to a lifestyle change.*** Losing weight permanently requires a commitment to changes . . . in your thinking, your lifestyle, your mind-set. It requires gaining knowledge and making permanent changes in your life for the better!

9. ***Thou shalt embrace the journey.*** This is a journey that will change your life; it's not a diet but a lifestyle! Be kind and supportive to yourself. Learn to applaud yourself for the smallest accomplishment. And when you slip up sometimes, know that it is okay; it is called being human.

10. ***Thou shalt live, love, and laugh.*** Laughter is still good for the soul. Live your life with passion! Never give up on your dreams! And most important . . . love! Remember that love never fails!

Now that you have experienced the power of healthy living, be sure to share your success story with others and help them to reclaim their health and vitality.

Appendix A

Quick Reference for JJ's Favorite Detox Products

DETOX METHOD	JJ'S FAVORITE BRAND	
Alkaline Water	IonPod	Kangen Machine
Chi Machine	Sun Ancon	
Colon Cleansing Herbs	Mag07	Colonix
Detox Foot Pads	BodyRelief	Asako
Apple Cider Vinegar	Bragg	
Liver Cleansing	Liver Rescue	Livatone

Appendix B

Guide to JJ's Online Communities

PROGRAM/ ONLINE COMMUNITY	SOCIAL MEDIA	PURPOSE	LINK
JJ's Private VIP Program	Facebook and Online Portal	Get hands-on support and coaching from JJ to help you accelerate your weight-loss results	https://www.jjsmithonline .com/products/healthy-new -black.html
10-Day Green Smoothie Cleanse Support Group	Facebook	Get support and encouragement from thousands who are currently doing the Green Smoothie Cleanse	https://www.facebook.com/ groups/Green.Smoothie .Cleanse/
JJ's Fan Page	Facebook	Join a community of over 1 million folks looking to lose weight and get healthy	https://www.facebook.com/ RealTalkJJ/
JJ's Instagram Account	Instagram	Be encouraged and inspired on your weight-loss journey through pictures	https://www.instagram.com/ jjsmithonline/?hl=en
JJ's Twitter Account	Twitter	Stay connected with JJ through her Twitter account	https://twitter.com/ JJSmithOnline
JJ's GSC Leaders	Facebook	Become a GSC Leader to help others successfully complete the 10-Day Green Smoothie Cleanse	https://www.jjsmithonline .com/products/gsc-certified -leadership.html

INDEX

About the Author

www.JJSmithOnline.com

JJ SMITH is a #1 *New York Times* bestselling author, nutritionist, and certified weight-loss expert, passionate relationship/life coach, and inspirational speaker. She has been featured on *The Steve Harvey Show, The View, The Montel Williams Show, The Jamie Foxx Show,* and *The Michael Baisden Show.* JJ has made appearances on the NBC, FOX, CBS, and CW Network television stations, as well as in the pages of *Glamour, Essence, Heart and Soul,* and *Ladies' Home Journal.*

Since reclaiming her health, losing weight, and discovering a "second youth" in her forties, bestselling author JJ Smith has become the voice of inspiration to those who want to lose weight, be healthy, and get their sexy back! JJ Smith provides lifestyle solutions for losing weight, getting healthy, looking younger, and improving your love life!

JJ has dedicated her life to the field of healthy eating and living. JJ's passion is to educate others and share with them the natural remedies to stay slim, restore health, and look and feel younger. JJ has studied many philosophies of natural healing and learned from some of the great teachers of our time. After studying and applying knowledge about how to heal the body and lose weight, JJ went on to receive several certifications—one as a certified nutritionist and another as a certified weight-management expert. JJ received her certification as Nutritionist from the Institute of Holistic Healing. JJ received her certification as a Weight-Management Specialist from the National Exercise and Sports Trainers Association (NESTA). She is also a member of the American Nutrition Association (ANA).

JJ's newest book, a #1 *New York Times* bestseller, *10-Day Green Smoothie Cleanse,* is a proven plan to safely and quickly detoxify the body, and jump-start weight loss. Most people who follow the plan strictly experience weight loss of up to 15 pounds in only ten days. JJ's last book, a #1 bestseller, *Lose Weight Without Dieting or Working Out!,* is a revolutionary system that teaches proven methods for permanent weight loss that anyone can follow, no matter their size, income level, or educational level. And the result is a healthy, sexy, slim body.

JJ holds a BA in mathematics from Hampton University in Virginia. She continued her education by completing The Wharton Business School Executive Management Certificate program. She served as vice president and partner in an IT consulting firm, Intact Technology, Inc., in Greenbelt, Maryland. JJ was also the youngest African American to receive a vice president position at a Fortune 500 company. Her hobbies include reading, writing, and deejaying.

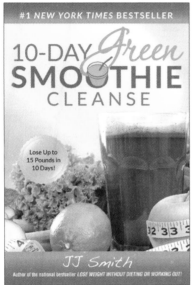
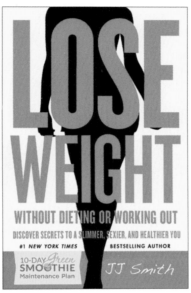
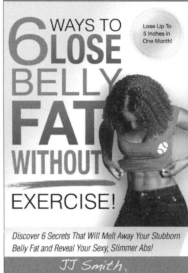
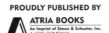